Alexandra Allred

PAS Fitness

Fitness for All

by Alexandra Allred

Copyright © 2016 by Alexandra Allred

All rights reserved. No part of this publication may be reproduced, distributed, or transmitted in any form or by any means, including photocopying, recording, or other electronic or mechanical methods, without the prior written permission of the publisher, except in the case of brief quotations embodied in critical reviews and certain other noncommercial uses permitted by copyright law.

The information in this book is meant to supplement, not replace, proper fitness training. Like any sport involving speed, equipment, balance and environmental factors, PAS Fitness poses some inherent risk. The authors and publisher advise readers to take full responsibility for their safety and know their limits. Before practicing the skills described in this book, be sure that your equipment is well maintained, and do not take risks beyond your level of experience, aptitude, training, and comfort level.

Cover Design by T.M. Franklin

Formatting Design by Lindsey Gray

IBSN: 978-1-941398-12-8

ACKNOWLEDGMENTS

To all those who were excluded or overlooked … now is your time to shine.
A very special thank you to Melissa and Michael Boler of Bridges Training Foundation, Navarro College, Tarelton State University and the amazing Dr. Kayla Peak. To Jon Yamamoto and Scott Goodwin of IDEAS, Inc., you opened up new possibilities. To the Main Street Gym, you opened up so many more things when you opened your doors to this special group of people.
And to my students, thank you for being the best teachers I ever had!

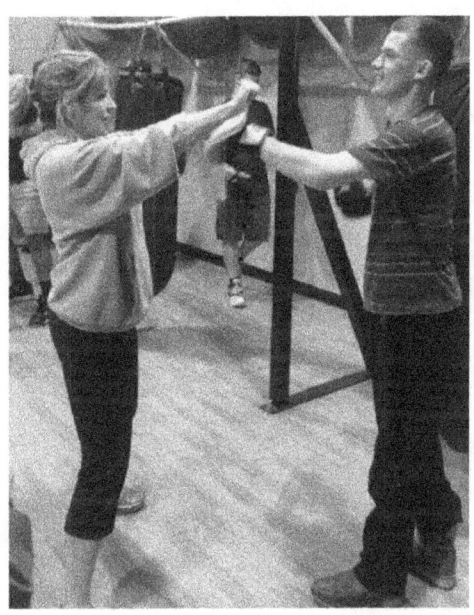

"No man has the right to be an amateur in the matter of physical training. It is a shame for a man to grow old without seeing the beauty and strength of which his body is capable."

~ Socrates

TABLE OF CONTENTS

Acknowledgments	i
Prelude: Personal Philosophy on Fitness and Training	Pg 1
Punch One: About PAS Fitness Training	Pg 3
Punch Two: The Athlete Within	Pg 9
Punch Three: What IS a Good Workout?	Pg 12
Punch Four: Working Your PAS Fitness System	Pg 16
Punch Five: Getting Started	Pg 19
Punch Six: Balance	Pg 35
Special Needs Facts: Who is Most Affected by Poor Balance?	Pg 37
Punch Seven: I CAN"T HEAR YOU!	Pg 42
Punch Eight: How to Move	Pg 45
Punch Nine: This Moves for You – How to Grow with PAS (πᾶς) Fitness	Pg 55
Punch Ten: Your Introduction to PAS Fitness and Empowerment	Pg 57
PAS Fitness Workout: Target	Pg 61
PAS Fitness Workout: Circuit	Pg 71
PAS Fitness Workout: Stability	Pg 83
Final Thoughts and Final Results of PAS Fitness	Pg 91
About the Team	Pg 94
Figures	Pg 97
Resources	Pg 99
About the Author	Pg 104

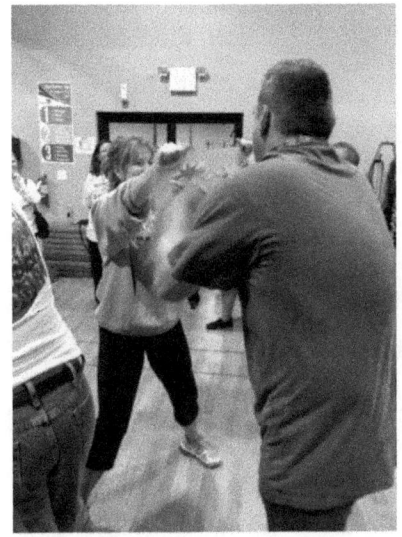

PRELUDE

Quite simply, this book came about because of an undeniable need.

In 2012, a class of special needs young adults was invited to participate in a regular kinesiology class at the Navarro College in Midlothian, Texas. The special needs class had been part of an "Elevate" program through the college in which students who had aged out of public schools could continue training and learning in hopes of one day earning a salaried job like their "normal" peers. The two instructors of each class had agreed that bridging a relationship between the two populations could be beneficial for all parties involved. They would have no idea how wonderful and powerful this idea would be!

Today, those two instructors are still working together to bridge relationships between the special needs and mainstream populations to debunk stereotypes, foster better understanding about the special needs community, and build a happier and healthier community.

Melissa Boler, founder of Bridges Training Foundation (www.bridgestf.org) and Alexandra Allred, creator of Pas Fitness have a dream to bring dignity, health, power, confidence, and education to every community across the nation and the world.

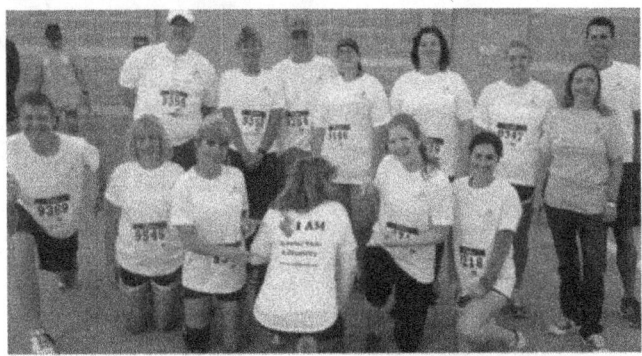

"The greatest barrier an individual with a disability will face is not their disability. But a society and the individuals it is made up of trying tell them what they are capable of achieving in their lifetime."

~ Melissa Boler

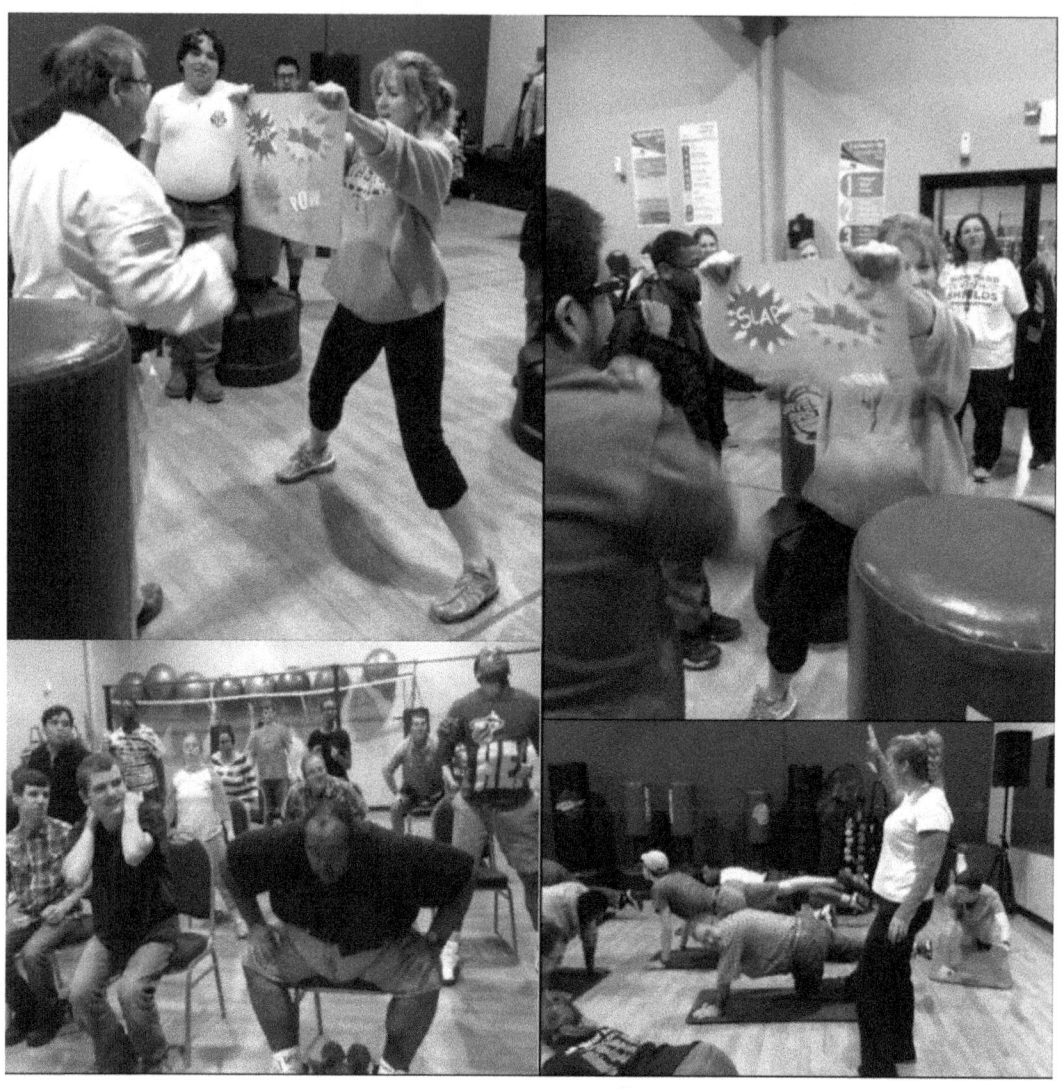

PAS FITNESS FOR EVERYONE!

PUNCH ONE
ABOUT PAS FITNESS

Who Can Do Pas Fitness Training?

-If you look at fitness DVDs and television programs, online workouts, and all the popular workout crazes today, who do you see? This is an easy answer. The vast majority of the exercise programs are directed exclusively toward 18 to 50+ year olds who are in reasonably good health and cardio condition.

-Sure. You see wonderful stories of extreme weight loss but the majority of the programs are geared toward people who can jump, perform burpees, push-ups, lunges and imitate speed skaters.

-What if you have a physical or developmental disability?
-What if you've had a knee replacement?
-What if you have balance issues?
-What if you cannot perform high impact moves due to a bad back or joints?
-What if you have foot problems or scoliosis?
-What if you are wheelchair bound? Or must use a chair during exercise?
-What if extra weight makes jumping and bounding not only dangerous but seemingly impossible?

-You are not alone!

What Are Special Needs?

-According to data compiled by the Center for Disease Control in Atlanta, the Census Bureau study in "Disability, Functional Limitation, and Health Insurance Coverage," the World Health Organization and the World Bank, approximately 800 million people live with significant physical or mental disability, including about 10 percent of children, in the world. In the United States, more than 75 million Americans live with some kind of physical or mental disability.

-Seventeen million people live with cerebral palsy but options for physical exercise are severely limited, not because of ability but because of lack of education and resources. Almost one million of these people are children, many of whom are looking for a physical outlet. And what about autism? There are more than four million Americans who live with autism spectrum disorder. It is the fastest-growing developmental disorder in the world. There is no known detection or cure and millions more will be affected by autism. Yet, when young adults "age out" of public school at age 22, their physical activity is greatly minimized. Specialized programs are extremely expensive.[1]

-Almost 20 million people report having difficulty walking a quarter-mile and nearly nine million simply cannot walk that distance. There are more than one million wheelchair users who both could and should find an exercise routine to keep muscles pliable, healthy and strong. Those who suffer from cystic fibrosis would benefit from punching to help break up the thick, sticky mucus that builds up on the lungs. And for the 20.5 million visually impaired Americans (120,000 of whom are completely blind)[2], and the 37 million who are legally blind across the globe, traditional exercise regiments are not only dangerous but seemingly impossible.[3]

The Growing Population of Seniors

By the year 2030, more than 72 million people (or approximately 20 percent of the U.S. population) will be over the age of 65. Today, of the nearly 40 million Americans over the age of 65, just 22 percent report being physically active on a regular basis. Beyond protection against high blood pressure, heart disease and diabetes, research has shown that exercise can also reduce the risk of certain cancers, increase lung capacity and better ensure bone density. With exercise comes more independence. When we exercise, we gain more mobility, more agility and stability. When we exercise, the brain is stimulated in a way that helps to prevent dementia, memory loss and depression.[4] Medical and long-term costs are greatly reduced for seniors who regularly exercise.

Weight Does Matter and Why You Should Care

For those who suffer from obesity, you already know the medical reasons you should exercise. You already know how hard it is to find an exercise program that is realistic and manageable for your joints/body. It can all be a bit daunting, but let's consider the medical reasons.

> • Obesity related medical treatments cost the United States between $150 to $210 billion annually.
> • Obesity related job absenteeism costs the U.S. $4.3 billion annually.
> • Hospitalizations for children and youth due to obesity related issues exceeds costs of $250 million annually.

---

[1] https://www.autismspeaks.org/what-autism/facts-about-autism
[2] http://www.afb.org/info/blindness-statistics/2
[3] http://timesofindia.indiatimes.com/india/India-has-largest-blind-population/articleshow/2447603.cms
[4] http://health.usnews.com/health-news/articles/2007/10/30/senior-citizens-need-to-work-out-too

> • Medical claims and hospitalization of obese employees has substantially changed medical costs to all Americans, including costs for new (larger) MRI equipment, beds, gurneys, ambulances, wheelchairs and other need medical equipment to fit larger people.[5]

Did you know that 10 pounds on fat on the stomach exerts 50 pounds of pressure on the spine? For so many suffering from chronic back pain, better health and fitness could help relieve that pain yet they are unable to do so without guidance.

Costs for children and adults with developmental and physical disabilities also come with burdensome price tags.

> • Children with Down syndrome have a medical cost 12 to13 times higher than a child without Down syndrome.[6]
> • The lifetime cost of caring for a child with autism is $1.4 million.
> • Costs for needed items such as wheelchairs, special beds, baths, walkers, even eating utensils have a price tag that is tripled that of a mainstream product.[7]

While these costs are certainly not fair, they are very real. In many cases, exercise can help to reduce (however minor) costs and improve health.

By exercising, you can build your aerobic capacity. This doesn't sound like much but when you age or become unhealthy, all that huffing and puffing you do just to walk up a slight incline is your body screaming for help. Believe it or not, exercise really is your friend. To reiterate, it helps to reduce high blood pressure, the risk of type 2 diabetes, and excess body fat while boosting your immune system and muscle mass. This is hugely important as we age. Exercise helps to keep the bones strong while reducing the risk of arthritis. Energy levels are raised, self-esteem is boosted, and confidence soars. You sleep better, you feel better, you look better! Research also shows that when you exercise, it raises your level of intelligence and memory. How about that?

For those with developmental and/or physical issues beyond the norm, however, there are added benefits. Because autism is the fastest-growing developmental disability in the world right now, let's use some research to illustrate a point.

Keeping in mind that there is a wide spectrum of disabilities and behaviors within the autistic diagnosis, exercise has proven to be very beneficial. Again, there are exceptions. For this reason, you must first speak to your personal physician before attempting any exercise routine. As previously discussed, when special needs young adults "age out" of public school, many are suddenly without a routine and exercise activities. Health suffers. The rise of obesity among children is already a global issue but for children and adults with medical and developmental issues, the risks are much greater. With weight issues come medical costs. Diabetes, cardiovascular disease, bone and joint problems, even

---

[5] http://stateofobesity.org/facts-economic-costs-of-obesity/
[6] http://www.cdc.gov/features/birthdefectscostly/
[7] http://www.thedailybeast.com/articles/2014/06/11/the-cost-of-raising-a-special-needs-son.html

depression all come with a price tag in addition to the emotional cost on the human being.

A number of studies involving structured exercise routines and individuals with autism revealed significant decrease in body mass, increased aerobic capabilities and better balance, agility, speed, strength, and flexibility.

Researchers have also found that some of the typical behaviors of those with autism, such as body rocking, head-nodding, self-talk, hand-flapping, tapping of objects, and pacing were better controlled when a structured exercise routine was introduced and maintained. Aggressive and self-injurious behaviors were decreased.

The Pas Fitness workout is beneficial in that it offers a routine that helps to improve attention span and improve motor skills while building confidence.[8] "We're awesome because we all have autism!"

What Is Pas Fitness Workout?

In the fitness industry, regardless of the activity, people are consistent on these levels:

- Most people do not like to leave their comfort zone.
- Most people believe they are working harder than they actually are.
- Most people believe they are perfectly mimicking their instructor, especially if they are sweating!
- And…many people will continue to perform the exact same function, despite correction after correction, because it feels better than the perfected form.

And that's in the gym or dojo, one-on-one with an instructor or trainer. If you are working out at home, how do you know how well you are performing? Chances are you are NOT working as hard as you think you are! Most people who work out at home honestly and truly believe they are kicking as high, squatting as deeply, punching as hard and leaping as high as the video instructor.

No, you're not!

So, How Can You Know?

The Pas Fitness workout is designed for seven purposes:

1. Aerobic stamina (however great or small – your choice)
2. Balance
3. Strength and muscle development
4. Coordination
5. Cognitive training
6. Self-esteem

---

[8] https://www.autismspeaks.org/science/science-news/sports-exercise-and-benefits-physical-activity-individuals-autism

7. Power

With the Pas Fitness workout, you can HEAR how hard you are working. With this design, you will raise your level and intensity and before you know it, will be punching and kicking harder than ever before.

People LOVE the sound of their powerful punches. It is very cathartic, it builds stamina, muscle development, and rhythm. Plus, let's face it…it's fun!

How Can You Grow?

The Pas Fitness workout is designed for EVERYONE! You do not have to be a 19-year-old athlete to challenge yourself. It is adjustable so anyone can use it. Sitting, standing, needing the assistance of a chair for balance, you CAN do this. Here's how:

You may not be able to lift your leg any higher than a few inches from the ground. The reality is this…if you are ambulatory but struggle with stepping up on a curb, taking stairs, stepping into a bathtub, this program is for you!

The "target" can be lowered to the ground, allowing even the most balanced- and hip flexion challenged person the opportunity to grow. Whether a partner holds the target or you use our Pas Fitness stand, adjust the target to the preferred height and document where the target is. If you began the Pas Fitness workout system for kicks at a 1.5, write it down. You may stay there for several weeks or months and that is okay but as you develop muscle, strength, endurance, coordination, and power, you WILL be able to raise the leg just a little higher and up goes the target. This is how you grow! This is how you can measure your own improvement.

Forget the scales. How strong you feel is so much more important!

Some students may have the target to the highest level, kicking Jackie Chan style with Arnold Schwarzenegger power while others position it at knee-length height. In Silver Sneakers, a class offered for active older adults with certified instructors through Healthways, where balance can be more of an issue, we never raise the foot above shin-level as the challenge is about balance and stability. In either case, however, being able to raise the knee or foot with confidence, strength, stability, and power is very important.

In punching, the rules still apply. How fun it is to see women who never threw a punch in their lives suddenly punching with certain power, working their backs, shoulders, and arms, streamlining muscles and developing the core!

And talk about confidence! When you hear how that target pops as you hit it, it will spur you on to go a little harder and a little faster each time.

How Can You Improve?

With the Pas Fitness workout, the unique measuring system and sound with which to measure your level of intensity allows you to document your progress. While an exerciser can know how well he or she is developing in other systems based on level of completion, what about form? What about intensity?

Rare is the person who gives 100 percent an entire exercise regimen. We ALL have peaks and valleys in our workouts. The more seasoned athletes know when they are dropping off in intensity but most people cannot feel this. They know simply that they are tired and, unwittingly, begin to slow down. Often times elite athletes will not realize how much they have fallen off their pace until they train against a clock or timer.

Similarly, in the Pas Fitnessworkout, you can HEAR and count how much you have slowed down. As it will be discussed later, this is when you simply document the slowing pace OR try to pick it up. Either way, you are measuring your results and it is exciting to watch as you grow over time.

The Pas Fitness workout is unlike anything else you've ever tried. Whether you are an elite athlete, a weekend warrior, a 65-year-old or older person, a person with some kind of developmental and/or physical disability, combating obesity, or working on balance issues, you will fall in love with this workout and what it can do for you long term.

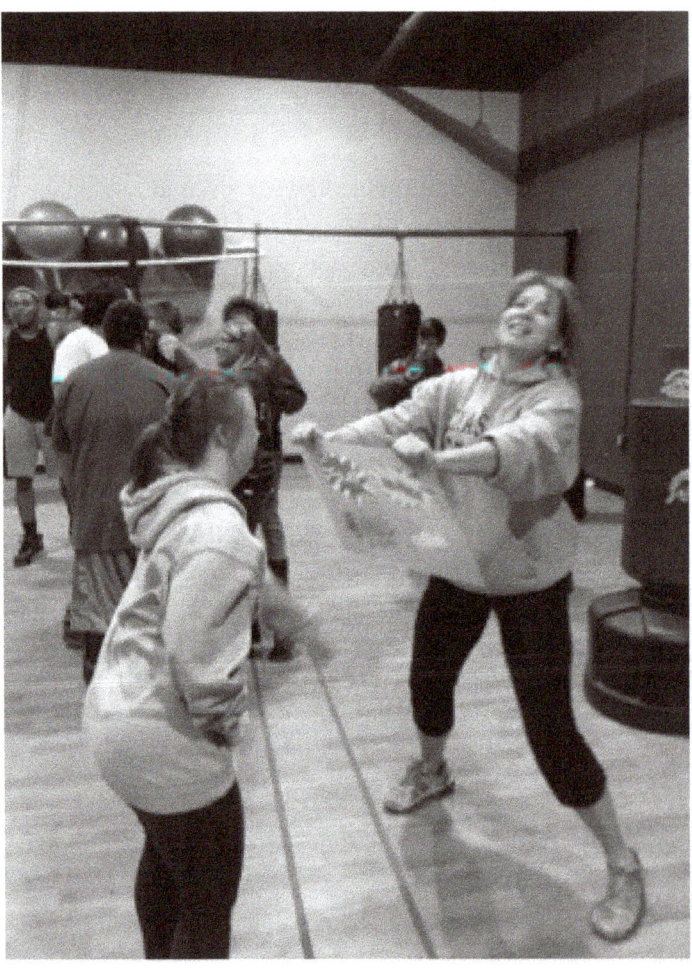

PUNCH TWO
THE ATHLETE WITHIN

What is an athlete?

Everyone has a picture in his or her mind of what a real athlete is, what they look like, how they act or move.

Following many of my classes, particularly if I have new people, I will ask:

Are you an athlete?

Nervous giggles.

Most people are very uncomfortable with idea of identifying themselves as an athlete. After all, an athlete is an obscenely overpaid professional who has dedicated himself or herself to a specific sport with great results. They exude confidence and have the muscles to show for it. Right?

That's just the showy part.

No, a true athlete is so much more. A true athlete is a person who strives to improve form, time, and strength. An athlete pushes to try a little harder, to get out of that comfort zone that MOST people "train" in, and an athlete doesn't quit the training session.

After a hard class, as we're all sprawled out on the floor – sweaty, exhausted, but content, I'll ask, "Are you an athlete?" but with a few more qualifiers:

Did you work your hardest?
Yes!
Did you quit?
No. I wanted to but I didn't quit.
Will you be back to do it all again?
Yes!
Do you have a goal in mind? Are you trying to improve you?
Yes!

Then comes that great moment. They realize, "Hey, I am an athlete." Discovering that athlete within is such a surprise to so many. But why? We sell ourselves short so often. We do not realize our own potential, how strong we are, how truly amazing we can be! The Pas Fitness workout – believe it or not – really does awaken that athlete within.

The punching and kicking WILL empower you and awaken that competitive spirit in you that makes you realize you ARE strong and can accomplish so much.

For nearly 30 years, I have taught countless men, women, boys and girls all shapes and sizes. I've worked with victims of domestic violence, physical assault, and rape. I've worked with people mending from knee, hip, and shoulder replacements, weak backs, seizures, and strokes. I've also had the tremendous honor of working with those with developmental, physical disabilities, weight and image issues.

How amazing it is to watch a person realize his or her own potential, to discover an inner strength they did not know they possessed, and exude a new sense of pride and self-worth. That's that inner athlete! Yes, punching and kicking really can do all that and safely. By using no- to low-impact exercises, this is an INCLUSIVE club that invites everyone to be challenged and grow.

It is time to stop selling yourself short. Don't believe all that you see when you look at other "athletes." As a former national and professional athlete, one who has lived half her life in a gym, I've watched as the "athletes" puffed around the training facilities. Every day I see men who can lift a refrigerator but could not run down the block to save his life. At a first muscled-glance, many would call him an athlete. But what would you call a middle-aged, slightly overweight woman who dutifully works out four times a week, never quits, always pushes, wants to succeed and better herself each day? An athlete!

Now it's your time!
Challenge yourself.
Don't quit.
Believe you are much stronger than you have given yourself credit for.
And if you have a bad workout…dust yourself off and strive for greatness again tomorrow.

Embrace your inner athlete!

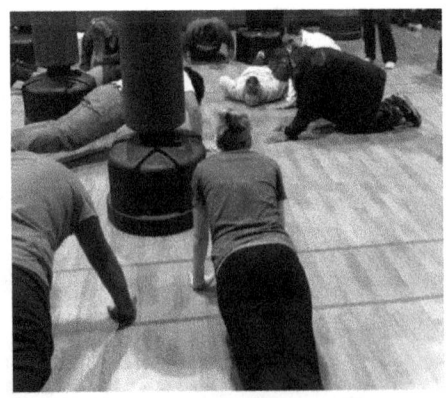

Throughout the weeks of training, one student wanted to do planks despite the fact that he lacked core strength ... but with practice and teammates cheering him on, he began to learn how to plank! Behind every athlete are great coaches, friends, and teammates! Which one are you?

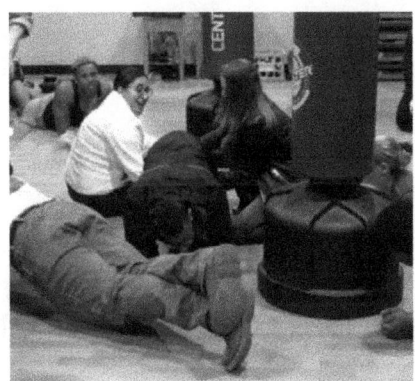

PUNCH THREE
WHAT IS A GOOD WORKOUT?

Do not exchange good form for time or weights!

Okay, what does that mean?

Instructors and trainers see this in the gym ALL THE TIME! A guy will come in and hammer out bicep curls, bench press and squats with big weights, lots of grunting and TERRIBLE form! When people give up form for higher or faster reps, they increase the chances of injury and minimize actual results.

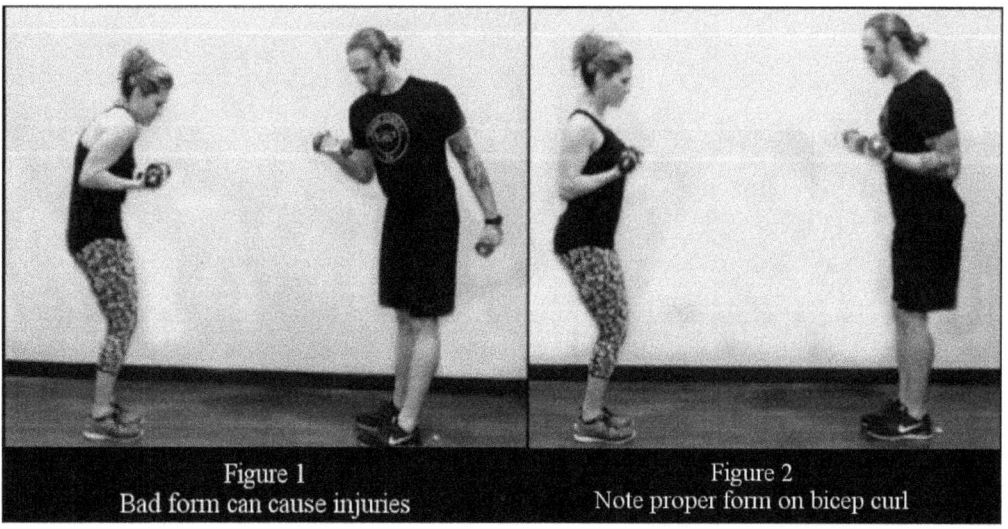

Figure 1
Bad form can cause injuries

Figure 2
Note proper form on bicep curl

In figure 1, note how Dionne's body is caving in because the weight it too heavy. Micah, on the right, is swinging his weight. His body is out of alignment. With each swing, his back is rotating and shoulders are unstable.

In figure 2, both trainers are strong. Note a slight bend in the knees, shoulders are drawn up and pulled back. The abdominals (core) is engaged and they are controlling – not swinging – the weights.

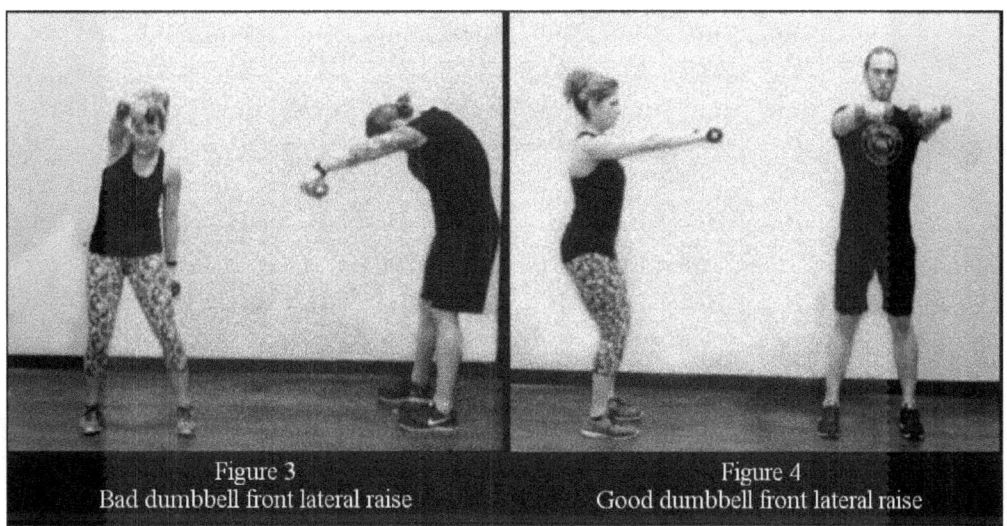

Figure 3
Bad dumbbell front lateral raise

Figure 4
Good dumbbell front lateral raise

In Figure 3, our trainers are not just being silly. These are positions we see in the gym on a daily basis yet most people have no idea this is what they are doing. Note how their heads are down, they are not controlling but swinging the weights, and their backs are compromised. Now check out the difference with Figure 4.

In Figure 4, their form is perfect. Each trainer has his or her head up, their core is engaged, back is strong, shoulders back, with a slight bend in the knees so that their shoulders and hips are in alignment with their ankles. Imagine you could draw a line from ankles up to the shoulders. They are in a nice straight line and not tipping forward. They are controlling their weights and truly working out the muscles they intend to work.

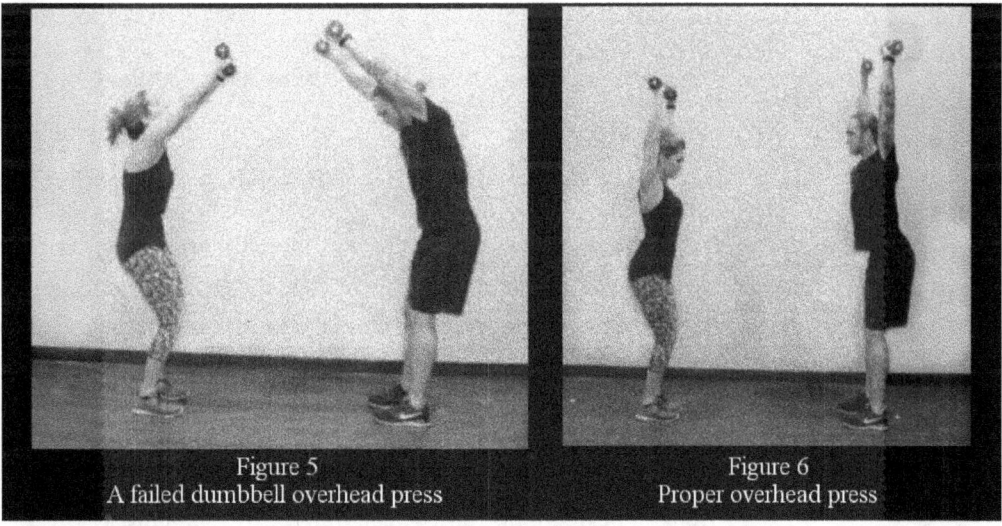

Figure 5
A failed dumbbell overhead press

Figure 6
Proper overhead press

In figure 5, note how both Dionne and Micah are collapsing with the weight. Dionne is looking up, losing focus/form while Micah is looking down and falling forward.

In figure 6, both trainers are looking straight ahead. They are focused. They are strong. There is a slight bend in the knees as the hips are locked over the ankles and back is straight.

KNOW THIS: Here are some very basic tips that fitness instructors and trainers would like you to think about while working out:

> • Focus on form. Your body IS your vehicle. Your body is your temple. Treat it well!
> • Work to exhaustion – that is, when you begin to lose form, end that set, rest, recover, try again!
> • Do not be afraid to push yourself!
> • Believe in yourself!
> • Think about proper alignment of your back
> • Keep your core strong

There is a fabulous article written by an up-and-coming coach from Tarleton State University, Coleman Furst, who discusses self-talk. While his focus is on playing sports, this great advice applies to working out in a fitness class or by yourself at home. Self-talk, those little thoughts and words that creep into your psyche, are incredibly powerful and WILL impact how and when you exercise.

Self-Talk: Whether You Think You Can or You Can't, You are Right

Nobody talks to you more than you do. All day long you have a subconscious running dialogue with yourself. What you think and what you say to yourself can have a great influence on your performance. You want to get to a place mentally in which you feel so internally positive that you can maintain a winning attitude through times of adversity during the game. The key is incorporating a sports psychology technique into your game preparation known as "self-talk," which can eliminate state anxiety and increase your self-confidence.

Self-talk can be described as the key to cognitive control as it refers to internal dialogue, including thought content and self-statements. It is up to you to decide if you are going to engage in negative or positive self-talk. For example, when you are in the heat of the game and you miss a shot, what do you say to yourself? If you are dwelling on the missed shot and the disappointment, you will most definitely lose self-confidence, anxiety control and concentration, all of which will certainly lead to poor performance. Like-wise, if you regain your composure and remind yourself of the countless shots you have made in practice every day, you will experience the opposite effect. Some of the reasons athletes employ negative self-talk are as follows:

> • Tuning in to errors so they can fix them, but then dwelling on them.
> • Being a perfectionist and setting unrealistic standards.
> • Engaging in all-or-nothing thinking ('I can't shoot') or over-generalization ('I always miss those shots').

It is important that you are aware of these dangerous thought patterns and instead shift to more positive thinking. It is easier said than done, but here are three action steps you can take to begin developing positive self-talk habits.

1. Choose a mantra

To get started with creating a more positive self-talk habit, choose one of two mantras you can use during your training. This could be a simple affirmation such as "I feel strong," or the mantra "I feel explosive," or another simple, positive phrase you can repeat over and over.

2. Practice multiple scenarios

Once you have developed the habit of repeating this phrase during practice to the point where it is automatic, start expanding the dialogue so that you have familiar and comfortable statements for a variety of situations during your sport. For example, after a missed shot in basketball you might say, "I'm a great shooter," or "next shot, best shot."

3. Create a positive mental image or visualization

The phrases and words you choose should be those that you can immediately call up and create a visual picture of yourself doing exactly what you say. The image along with the words are a powerful combination that creates a positive message tied to a belief.

Practicing this sort of sports psychology skill is one way to take your athletic performance to the next level.

What is your mantra?
- I deserve this!
- I will walk a mile!
- I will hold my grandchild!
- I will lose weight!

What are your multiple scenarios and are you ready for them?
- What will I say if someone tells me I can't do this?
- How will I react if I don't have a good workout?
(Psst – hint: Try again tomorrow!)
- What if someone laughs at me?

Most importantly, what mental images have you created for you and your future?
- A stronger you!
- A more confident you!
- A slimmer and trimmer you!
- Better balance!
- A happier you!

PUNCH FOUR
WORKING YOUR PAS FITNESS WORKOUT

The entire principle behind this workout routine is to introduce you to a stronger and more functional movement so that you can become more independent and confident in life. It will work your balance, coordination, control, agility, speed, and endurance. It is challenging but you CAN DO THIS!

What It Really Does

Earlier, we mentioned the Pas Fitness workout is designed for very specific purposes:

Aerobic Stamina:

As you learn to punch and kick, those movements will become more powerful and more effective as you practice. Quite simply, the more you do it, the stronger and better you will feel.

Every week, as someone new wanders into our Pas Fitness classes, the question is asked: "This feels awkward, doesn't it? Do you feel uncoordinated?" Invariably, the person always says, "Yes!" But that same person – always – only gets faster, stronger, and more precise if s/he continues to come to class. Time and practice really are your friends!

As your stamina builds, you become a more efficient machine. You sweat more. You burn more calories. You work harder and begin to see and feel the results over time.

Balance and Coordination:

Simply put, the sports definition of balance is to have the ability to stay upright or stay in control of body movement, and coordination is the ability to move two or more body parts under control, smoothly and efficiently.

Those most affected by imbalance are the special needs and senior citizen populations but balance is something everyone should work on all the time. Your balance can never be too good!

Strength and Muscle Development:

Each time you punch and kick, you build strength and muscle development. As you are punching and kicking, however, you're only thinking, WHY IS THIS SO HARD?

Why? As you are punching and kicking, it causes a kind of exhaustion or trauma of the cellular proteins in your muscle. Say what? Here's how it works: The breakdown of cellular proteins creates cell-signaling messages to awaken satellite cells that begin a complicated muscle repair and growth process. From there, the body reacts to the process and away your muscles grow![9] It sounds so confusing so remember this: As you exercise, the muscle growth you hope for will not occur during the exercise but when you rest. Work out, be the athlete you always wanted to be, challenge yourself and then rest!

While the process of building muscle is almost immediate after exercise, it may take weeks to months for you to see the change. But just because you don't see it, doesn't mean it is not happening. It is!

Cognitive Training:

What is cognitive training anyway? Cognitive thinking is the set of all mental abilities and processes related to memory, attention, knowledge, judgment and reasoning, problem solving and decision making. As this relates to physical activity, a person must use cognitive training to process and interpret how to move, react, and counteract. Learning balance, flexion, standing, sitting, catching a ball, or throwing a punch is all part of cognitive training.

A fascinating study, in which the brains of healthy subjects and of brain-damaged patients who had difficulty controlling movements were evaluated to determine two amazing things:

> 1. There are several regions in the brain collaborate that enhance or allow for more detailed motor action.
> 2. Practice really does make perfect. Okay, no one is perfect but it certainly improves things.

The study showed that because athletes are always accessing and using these regions of the brain, they are tapping into and conditioning greater cognitive skills. Every time an athlete mastered a new skills set or learned new patterns, the brain's communication train works just a little bit better. As we will discuss later on, each time you move, you are working numerous muscles. Your body is a machine!

As you work, brain neurons strengthen connections to one another using the front of the brain. That region, the prefrontal cortex, is the control panel that allows us to focus on a task or skill and weigh how to move or respond appropriately. As we practice, this region of the brain becomes more and more efficient and our reaction response quickens, making us better, faster, stronger. Even better? When we do cognitive training, the brain continues to change (or improve) for months.[10][11]

---

[9] https://www.unm.edu/~lkravitz/Article%20folder/musclesgrowLK.html
[10] http://discovermagazine.com/2010/apr/16-the-brain-athletes-are-geniuses#.UsFzLXazKpg
[11] Joe Vennare on 1/10/2014 Daily Burn. http://dailyburn.com/life/tech/brain-training-sports/

Self-Esteem:

Self-esteem is the natural by-product of improved cognitive state, of better balance and coordination, and of increased stamina. When you move better, you feel better. When you feel stronger, you feel more empowered. With improved balance and posture comes an improved attitude and before you know it, you are standing taller. You are more confident. Suddenly, you BELIEVE you can do things you once thought improbable or even impossible.

Finally, comes the **Power**.

Now, you may ask why 'power' came behind self-esteem. Wouldn't having more power improve a person's self-esteem? Perhaps. But on this building block, experience has proven again and again that when a person begins a strong punching and kicking program and begins to feel (and see) the results of better stamina, balance, coordination and cognitive training, that self-talk and self-esteem build. "I can do this!" "I am strong."

In the sports world, power is defined as explosive power, maximum exertion of strength within short bursts of movement. Like punching and kicking.

But that power, that ability to explode, to exert, to burst forward is truly a combination of everything explained in this chapter. Power is balance. Power is stamina, strength and muscle development. Power is cognitive thinking and power is self-esteem. You CAN achieve power.

PUNCH FIVE
GETTING STARTED

How to Punch

1-2-1-2 Punches

    Imagine you are sitting on a horse. If you have a workout buddy or someone who can look at your position, use them. Don't be shy. Ask for someone to look at how you are lined up before you begin punching to ensure you have the correct form.

- Feet are shoulder width apart, toes pointing forward. Make sure you don't allow your toes to point outward. We call those duck feet. Likewise, don't allow your toes to point inward. We call those pigeon toes.
- Shoulders are drawn back, chin up and have a slight bend in your knees. Here's where your training buddy or friend comes in. Ask them: Are my shoulders, hips and ankles in alignment?
- When you punch, one hand is out (punching) while the other is pulled back against your chest/rib cage. The punch fist is palm down with your first two knuckles hitting the target and the withdrawn hand is palm up.

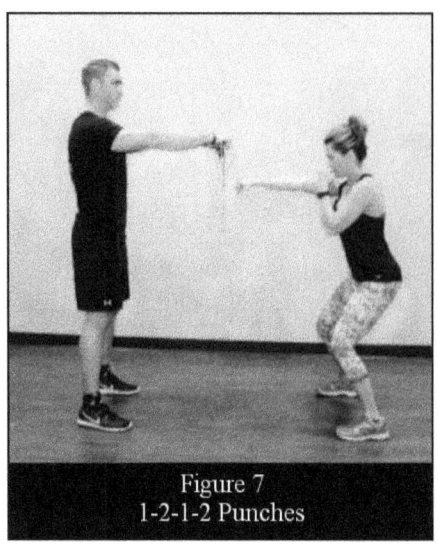
Figure 7
1-2-1-2 Punches

You might ask, why the positioning of the hands matter. Here's why:

This motion does three things at once. It works on form, full arm and back development, and it works cardio.

More importantly, learning to protect yourself is also important. In kickbox and boxing classes, students should be reminded to bring the hands back "to form" (that is, fists on either side of the face). Why? By doing so, you have a straight back, strong abs but you are also guarding your rib cage, abs and face by keeping the guards (or hands) up.

Proper Form

When you slow yourself down and properly position your fist while punching, it greatly improves your form. All too often (women more so than men), when people begin punching the target, they turn what could be a great workout into a half-workout in which muscles are shortened, cardio is limited and not to mention, sissy-punching.

The sissy punch is when both hands are fisted and kept right in front of the chest. While one fist is striking the target, the other remains in front of the chest GREATLY reducing range and power. The result is more of a flicking of the wrists and fists than hard landing punches.

Picture you and your little sister when you are eight years and six years old, facing turned to the side, eyes squeezed shut and swinging wildly at each other. Voila! The sissy punch.

The full punch is when the left hand lashes out with great power to hit the target, the right hand is withdrawn, palm inward, against the side of your face or jaw. As soon as you begin to withdraw the left (punching) hand, the right hand punches out with full extension and explosive power. As the right hand lands on the target, the left hand is pulled back, fist rotating so that the palm inward against the side of the face or jaw.

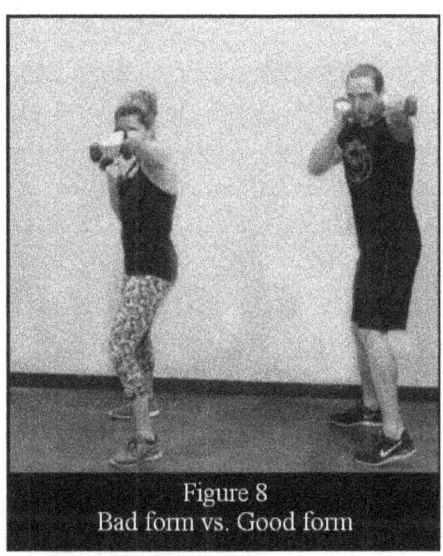
Figure 8
Bad form vs. Good form

In Figure 8, note how Dionne has a little bit of the sissy punch going. Her punching hand (left hand holding weight) is dropped. Her shoulders are dropped forward ever so slightly. Now look at Micah on the right. His left punch is solid! His wrist is not bent but strong, forming a long, strong line to his target.

It's all a habit! So, slow the pace down until you get this motion. What ALWAYS happens is that the puncher gets very excited about the power, the punching, the thrill of it all and forgets form.

When you have done this over and over, having thrown hundreds of punches, it does imprint in your brain and before you know it, you are throwing perfect punches but until that time, slow down the pace, make sure the punching fist is palm down and the withdrawn fist is pulled all the way back with palm up.

Arm and Back Development

Looking at the two pictures, you can already see the difference in how the arms and back are worked simply by looking at the positioning of the hands. The (incorrect) hands pulled up toward the chest limit the range of the punch, thus limiting the development of the arm and back muscles. Instead of developing longer and leaner muscles, you are half-ing that motion.

When the punches are thrown at full extension and the hand/fist turns over (palm down) while the retracting hand/fist comes back (palm up), this constant changing of hand positioning works the tricep and bicep muscles beautifully. The action demands that you, the puncher, have greater form and generate more power.

This full range power opens up your back, utilizing the trapezius, teres minor, teres major, and dorsi muscles. This is a fabulous workout for the deltoid, pectoralis major muscles as well. It is important to understand that when you use this proper form, you are engaging multiple muscles groups to build a better, stronger, more complete body.

Cardio

With this proper form, the back and lungs are opened up and with proper hand placement, your cardio work goes up. When the hands are at chest level or higher, your heart works harder. This is true for other activities too, such as walking. The American Council on Exercise notes that your caloric expenditure and oxygen intake increases while engaged in activities such as punching.

KNOW THIS: Many people unknowingly drop the punches lower, below heart rate level. This reduces your cardio work, not to mention diminishes form.

KNOW THIS: Dionne and Micah are punching with weights in Figure 8 but you do NOT have to use weights when you begin this workout program. We recommend beginning with no- to very light weights as your body becomes acclimated to this new routine.

Single Jabs

In boxing, it is the back hand that is the power punch but in kickbox it is opposite. We use the front or forward hand just as we use the front or forward leg which is where the surprise and power lies. Again, this is why balance is so essential. To repeat: Use your side that is facing toward the target. When we discuss the jab and roundkick combination, it is always the front side unless otherwise specified ("back jab" or "back leg roundkick"). Kickbox and martial arts is the platform for the Pas Fitness workout, which uses same side action.

Let's use the left single jab as our example.

- With the left foot forward, body turned to the side, and both fists up, you are ready to start. Place your fist on either side of your chin/jawbone.
- The rules still apply. As you punch, the hand turns over so that the palm it down and you are hitting with knuckles one and two.
- As soon as you hit, immediately retract the punch back to the side of your face.

This is for two reasons:

1. When you immediately bring the striking hand/fist back to the side of the face, you are learning to stand in "fight mode." You are protecting the side of your face – important fighter stance – that enables you to have better form. When the hand is allowed to drop, so do the shoulders.
2. With the hands up over the heart, you increase your cardio and stamina.

Bonus result: Again, this is all habit. But once you get into the habit of bringing those fists back to the sides of your face, people report feeling "like a fighter!" Self-esteem and great workouts with great results all go hand in hand. It taps into the athlete within!

So don't drop those hands.

Got it?
Now try the other side.

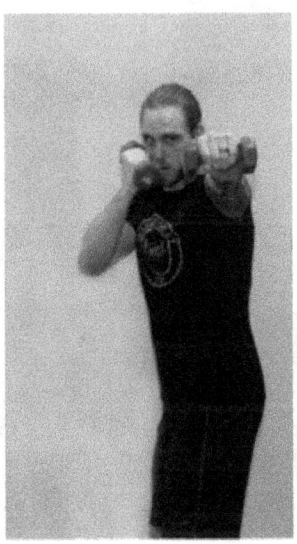

Hooks

The exact same principles apply as it did with the single jab. If you are throwing a hook punch with your right hand, the right foot is forward. Both hands/fists are drawn up alongside your face and you almost ready to go.

The hook, unlike the punch that shoot straight out, is just what it sounds like. It is a hooking motion for a punch.

-Let's use the right hook punch for the example:

> • Palm facing downward, the power generates from your right shoulder.
> • Stand sideways to the target.
> • Imagine you are beginning to push something out to the side of you (with tremendous power) and then you hook it around to the front of you.
> • As soon as the hand/fist is back to the side of your face, strike again. The movement should be quick and powerful.
> • This is a power movement that comes from the shoulder, back and abdominals.

With everything you do with this program, you need to understand what muscles are being engaged so you can better appreciate how hard you are working and how amazing your body truly is.

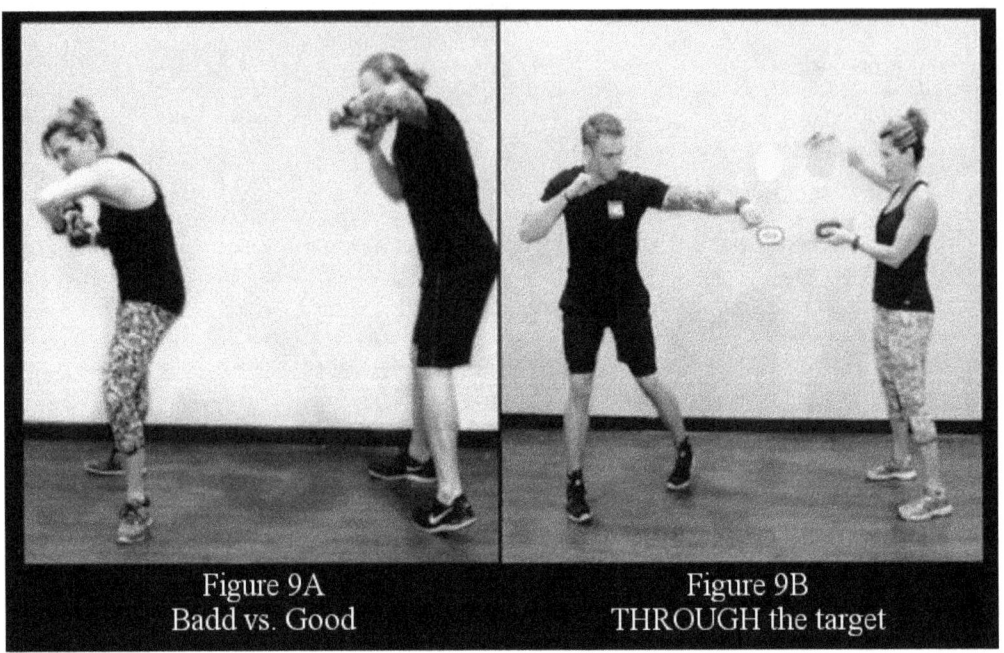

Figure 9A
Badd vs. Good

Figure 9B
THROUGH the target

Note how Dionne is folding in or collapsing inward with the punch. *Also note how her left foot is turned out. On the right, Micah's hook is strong. Elbow is level to his fist, chin or nose level, and as he throws the hook technique, see how he puts his left hip into it. Note how his left heel follows in line with his hip.

How to Bob and Weave

Whether you are performing a series of punches, upper cuts or kicks, the bob and weave is designed for two reasons: evade and explode.

You see boxers bob and weave all the time. You've probably even pretended to be a "contender," simulating a boxer, playfully dancing around your invisible opponent.

Practice in the mirror. Imagine that someone throws a punch at you. You – with fists on either side of your face – duck, shuffle side to side, jump a half-set back and then lunge forward, then shift back in a power stance to shuffle (dance) side to side.

The key points to a bob and weave is:

- Place one foot forward. Example: right foot.
- Place fists at "guard position" – on either side of your jaw line.
- With the right foot forward, your right hand should be slightly higher on the guard position since it is closest to your real or imagined opponent. This guard hand can cover the entire side of your head.
- The left guard hand is furthest from your opponent. That fist is dropped to the jawline in case a roundhouse kick or hook should swing around in

an attempt to catch your jaw and knock you out. I know, I know…this isn't real but it is important for you to understand WHY your hands and feet are in the position that they are! Right now you ARE a boxer/kickboxer. Let's tap into that athlete within!

• In the split stance, shift your weight onto the balls of your feet. Do not stand flat footed. On the balls of your feet, you can move more easily and quickly from side to side, forward and backward. This is your offense and defense – the bob and weave.

1-2-1-2 Upper Cuts

You are back on the horse again! Facing toward the target, imagine you are back in the saddle, fists drawn and ready to go. The stance is very similar to the 1-2-1-2 punches:

• Feet are shoulder width apart, toes pointing forward. Make sure you don't allow your toes to point inward or outward. Remember pigeon toes and duck feet.
• Shoulders are drawn back, chin up, and have a slight bend in your knees. Here's where your training buddy or friend comes in. Ask them: Are my shoulders, hips, and ankles in alignment? Chin up?
• Fists drawn, deliver short, power punches with the palm turned upward!
• Here comes the bob and weave! It is very hard to generate power (especially for females) without moving the feet and hips on the upper cut punch.

Let's look at the bob-and-weave. As you get more advanced, you will feel quite comfortable with the bob and weave as you punch but at the beginning, it may feel awkward. That's okay. Practice, practice, practice. This is all about developing skills that become so natural to you that you won't even realize how much you are moving as you punch and kick. As we learn new techniques, standing still is to be expected but we are limited in power on the upper cuts as it is a short-action punch. It is difficult to generate power while standing still so adding a bend to the knee and thrusting upward with some hip action definitely helps.

The idea is to "load up," that is, retract the fists to either side of your face, at the jaw line. In essence, you are protecting your jaw or the side of your face in order to (you hope) block a blow.

Let's start with your left side as an example of technique and explosion:

• As you ready to throw a left upper cut, the left shoulder drops.
• As the left shoulder drops so, too, does the left fist as it will be exploding upward.
• Left fist rolls upward – palm up.
• Explode/thrust upward WITH hip thrust. Here comes that bob and

weave again!

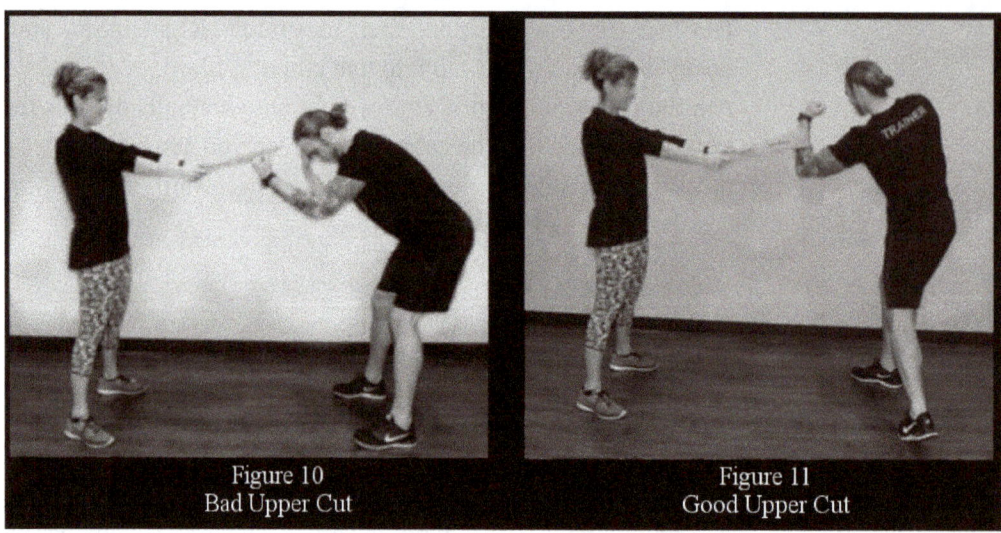

Figure 10
Bad Upper Cut

Figure 11
Good Upper Cut

The set up:

- When your left shoulder drops, so does your stance (the bob or mini squat).
- As soon as you throw the upper cut, explode upward, using power from your hip.

In Figure 10, notice how Micah has lost his form and focus. He is looking down and the power to his punches (upper cuts) will be minimized.

In Figure 11, he is using his hips to explode upward as he delivers an upper cut. See how his left foot and hip are pivoted into the punch, working with his upper body and maximizing full force. His head is up and he is watching the target!

Voila! The upper cut.

KNOW THIS: If you simply stand flat-footed, you greatly minimize power. Power comes from the hip in this motion.

How to Kick

You only THOUGHT you knew how to kick!

It is always easy to spot the former soccer players or dancers when they begin kickboxing. Soccer players love to wind up for the big kick and dancers are seasoned toe-pointers but in martial arts/ kickbox/ Pas Fitness Training, we have to put you somewhere in the middle.

KNOW THIS: If you were kicking something solid with a pointed toe, this could cause serious damage to your ankle. Fortunately, your target is light and flexible but think "strong ankle" as you kick. As you kick, you are working multiple muscles to build a stronger YOU. This includes balance.

Once you learn how to properly kick, you will be amazed how strong you become. Proper form with kicking teaches balance and confidence, but you will also engage abdominal muscle, lower back, hip, hip flexion, glutes, quads, hamstrings, ankles and instep (yes, you have muscle that needs to be worked on the arch of your foot!). This is what makes punching and kicking such a tremendous workout.

Front Kick

With the front kick, you face your target:

- Fist drawn up to either side of your face. Why? Two reasons:
    1. With fists up for each and every kick, it becomes habit. This habit is most important is self-defense. While you are exercising, learning why we do what we do in martial arts/kickboxing/Pas Fitness and embrace the self-protection of the art.
    2. Balance. Most people wave their hands and arms around while kicking and look like they are trying to help land an airplane. Don't land an airplane.
- Stand straight. Posture is very important. Chin up, shoulders back.
- Using the left leg as the example leg: Draw up the left knee, fists still on either side of the jaw line, pull the toes back toward the knee. This is called a Dorsey flex. This works the foot, ankle, knee, quad and hamstring with the opposite leg (your support leg) flexing hip, glutes, lower back, and abdominal muscles while fighting for balance.
- With toes pulled back, kick out. The ball of your foot should strike the target.
- Maintain good/strong posture with a straight back, immediately fold the foot back again after the kick, or the strike, and set down.

KNOW THIS: The front kick is a 4-point kick: Knee up, kick out, foot back (with bent knee again), and set down.

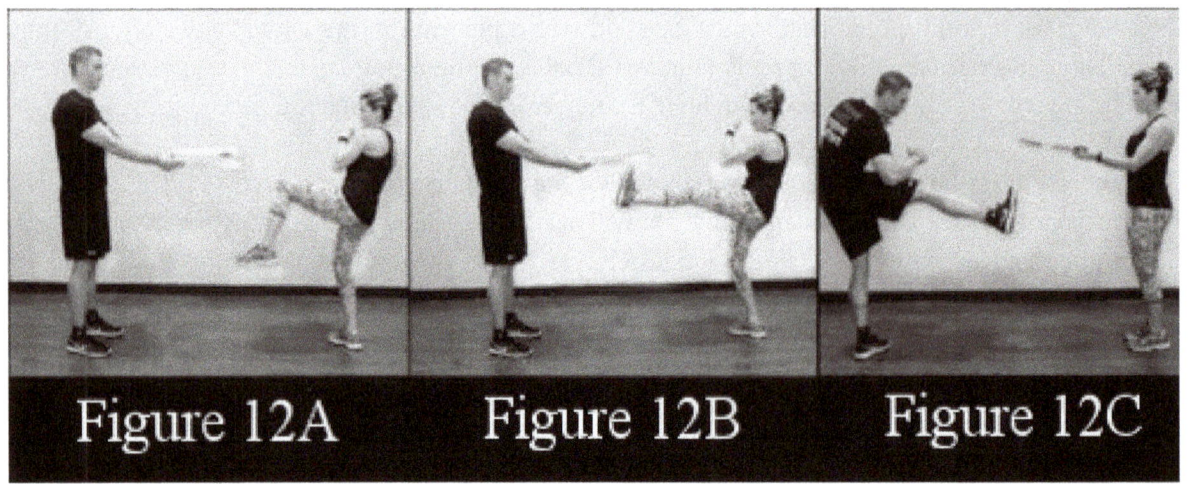

Figure 12A   Figure 12B   Figure 12C

Note in Figure 12A that Dionne is standing upright, guards (fists) are up and she is raising her knee up, steadying her balance to kick. In Figure 12B, she remains upright with a strong back and guards are up.

Dionne performed a perfect 4-point kick: knee up, kick out, pull foot back with a bent knee, and foot set down.

Below, however, in Figure 12C, Micah collapses forward into his front kick and loses form.

The purpose for the front kick is to push someone (bad guy) off of you. Using explosive power, the kick can throw the opponent backward and off balance to allow you time to run! In Pas Fitness workouts, this explosive kick works multiple muscles and balance. With hands up at the jawline, it will also increase your heartrate and cardio workout. Plus…it's fun!

KNOW THIS: You ARE a mean machine! You are tapping into that athlete within. You are NOT a member of the Rockettes! So remember, knee up, kick, snap the foot back, and set down. Do not kick as high as you can. Control! Control the kick. When you kick too high, you lose form and the shoulders will collapse forward.

Round Kick

With the front kick, you face your target. With the round kick, also known as a roundhouse kick, you stand sideways.

Here are the differences between a front kick and a round kick:

Front Kick	Round Kick
Face opponent or target	Stand sideways to opponent or target
Kicking leg: toes are pointed upward. Toes are pulled back so that striking surface is the ball of the foot.	Kicking leg: foot/toes are sideways. This means your hip is rotated over so naturally turns the foot sideways.
Support leg: power generated from the glutes.	Support leg: power is generated from the hips/glutes.

Note in Figure 12A that Dionne is standing upright, guards (fists) are up and she is raising her knee up, steadying her balance to kick. In Figure 12B, she remains upright with a strong back and guards are up.

Dionne performed a perfect 4-point kick: knee up, kick out, pull foot back with a bent knee, and foot set down.

Below, however, in Figure 12C, Micah collapses forward into his front kick and loses form.

The purpose for the front kick is to push someone (bad guy) off of you. Using explosive power, the kick can throw the opponent backward and off balance to allow you time to run! In Pas Fitness workouts, this explosive kick works multiple muscles and balance. With hands up at the jawline, it will also increase your heartrate and cardio workout. Plus…it's fun!

KNOW THIS: You ARE a mean machine! You are tapping into that athlete within. You are NOT a member of the Rockettes! So remember, knee up, kick, snap the foot back, and set down. Do not kick as high as you can. Control! Control the kick. When you kick too high, you lose form and the shoulders will collapse forward.

Round Kick

With the front kick, you face your target. With the round kick, also known as a roundhouse kick, you stand sideways.

Here are the differences between a front kick and a round kick:

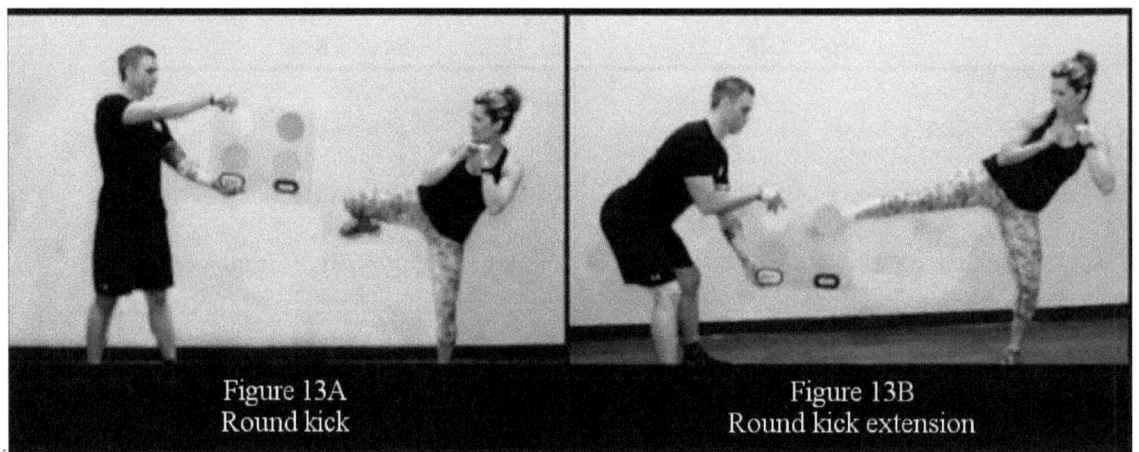

Figure 13A
Round kick

Figure 13B
Round kick extension

KNOW THIS: This requires balance! The higher you raise the knee; the more balance is required. This also puts pressure on the right hip, lower back, glute, and quad. Suddenly, all your weight has shifted to the right side of your body.

In Figure 13A, note how Dionne's guards are up and her core (her abdominals) are engaged. She has steadied her balance and only then draws her foot up.

In Figure 13B, she extends the kick, still holding her balance and her guards remain in place!

Also note that Micah has lowered the target in Figure 13B. While Dionne could easily kick higher, not everyone can kick high and certainly not beginners. Do not be in a rush to kick higher that what feels natural! You are in training so listen to your body.

It is a challenging kick because it is unnatural! Your entire life you walked, climbed stairs, ran, cycled, swam, used the Elliptical and/or treadmill moving in a forward motion. Now you are being asked to perform a sideways kick.

New muscle is being called upon.

- Standing sideways, left guard still up, left knee up, left foot pulled back to glute, kick out. The kick should extend fully to the target, pull the foot back again to the glute and set down.
- This is also a 4-point kick: Foot pulled back/knee up, kick out, snap it back, set foot down.

The Big DON'T of Round Kicks!

- No wind up! Here come the soccer players! This kick is about control. nEach time you kick and set the foot back down again on the floor, set the kicking leg back down in front of you. It is your "lead" leg. Do not allow it to swing back behind you. This is very bad for your back and hips, and is also bad form.

• By keeping the lead kicking lead in front, raising it up/kicking and setting it back down, you work proper form, engaging lower back, abdominals, hips, glutes efficiently and safely.

ADVANCED KICK
Outside Crescent Kick
ADVANCED KICK

The outside crescent kick IS an advanced kick. It works the entire core, back, glutes, hips, and legs – both kicking and support leg. But because of the shift in your stance, it can be very challenging for those with balance issues and/or weaker core/back.

What is the Outside Crescent?

To truly appreciate HOW to perform this kick, understand WHY this kick is used. From a self-defense perspective, this is a kick that can save you from a weapon. A bad guy is holding a weapon to you. You feel defenseless. What can you do? Using the outside crescent kick, you can kick the weapon away and run!

The key to this kick is explosive power and element of surprise. As soon as the knee comes up, you are committed to this kick! For surprise (and power) be ready to explode. Just as fast as the knee comes up, the leg straightens again and bursts out to the side with the outside of your foot hitting the weapon and knocking it away.

Like the front kick, the outside crescent kick is performed facing the target. Let's mix it up and use the right leg as the example striking leg:

• Stand straight. Posture is everything!
• Both guards are up, shoulders back, chin up.
• Slightly shifting weight to the left side, pick up right foot.
• With a slight bend in the right leg, draw the knee up (very slightly).
nSee picture*

1. Right leg prepares for kick. Note slight bend in knee.
2. Leg/knee moves inward, preparing leg for extension and burst out to the right.
3. Leg extends. Foot kicks out to the right with outside of right foot making contact with target.
4. The full motion is a large circle motion with the foot coming back down to the floor IN FRONT of you!

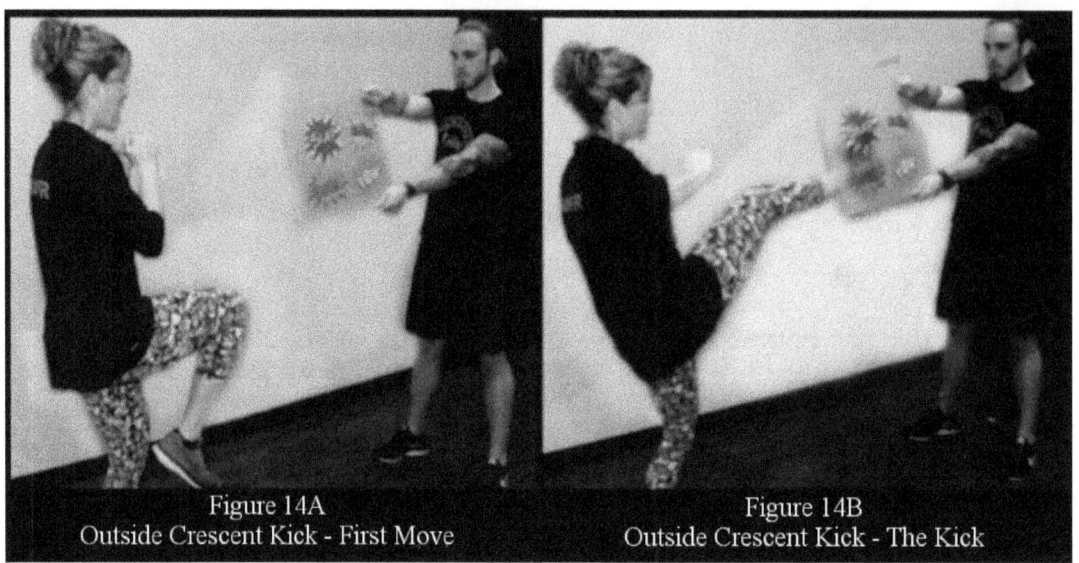

Figure 14A
Outside Crescent Kick - First Move

Figure 14B
Outside Crescent Kick - The Kick

In figure 14A, note how straight Dionne's back is. On this drill, her right leg is kicking leg so she draws up the right knee.

In figure 14B, as she draws that right knee up, she prepares to "explode" outward, straightening the leg and powering through the paper. In this move, the outside of Dionne's right foot slaps through the target.

What you don't see: As soon as Dionne's foot goes through the target, she will set it down in *front* of her to prepare to kick again – not behind her.

KNOW THIS: Just as there is no wind up for the round kick, do not wind up for the outside crescent kick. This is a powerful kick that must be controlled. When the foot starts and finishes in front of you, you engage your entire core (abdominal wall), lower back and legs. Fantastic! Woo! Here comes the athlete within!!

ADVANCED KICK
Hook Kick
ADVANCED KICK

Standing sideways, this begins like the roundhouse kick. With the round kick, the kicking leg/foot is sideways with the toe leading into the kick. With the hook kick, also standing sideways, the kick pulls backward so that the heel of the striking leg makes contact with the target.

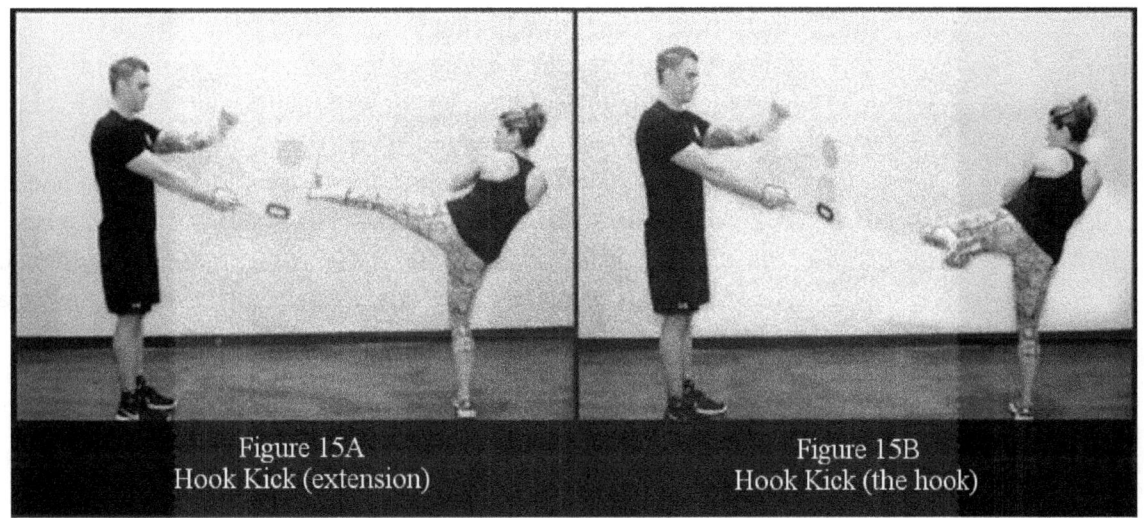

Figure 15A
Hook Kick (extension)

Figure 15B
Hook Kick (the hook)

In Figure 15A, Dionne extends her kick in front. Remember, this kick begins with you standing sideways (but also standing directly in front of the target) and guards are up. Note how her foot is sideways – hips turned to the side.

In figure 15B, she snaps the heel back. Note how her foot is turned so that her heel leads through the target.

Here are the differences between a round kick and a hook kick:

Round Kick	Front Kick
Standing Sideways	Standing Sideways
Kicking leg: power is generated from the hip flexor as knee pulls back and foot explodes forward.	Kicking leg: power is generated from the lower back and glutes as knee draws up toward chest and foor stikes backwards.
Contact of foot: toe or ball of foot	Contact of foot: heel

Again, balance is the name of the game. Standing sideways, using the right leg as the example kicking leg, place left hand on a rail, back of a chair or wall for balance. Here we go:

- Right guard is up to the jaw line, stand straight, shoulders back.
- Since we are using the right leg as the kicking leg, turn the toes of your left foot slightly toward the chair or wall that is your support base. This helps keep your foot/knee and hip in better alignment for the kick.
- Draw the right knee in toward the chest (slightly), extend leg and snap the kick backward. Many call this a "donkey kick."
- Be sure that the target is directly in line with your hip/side, shoulder. The real work is then being able to bring the knee in, extend the leg and kick backward through the target.
- Connect heel to target.

You are working balance, core, lower back, hips, abductors and adductors (inner and outer thighs)! Because you are working such large muscles, this is a heavy load on the lower back so gradually build. Do not try to kick too high or too fast too quickly.

Work on balance. Slowly develop stronger ab- and adductor muscles so that you can lift and hold the leg a little higher as time (and practice) go by. You have all the time in the world so take your time and work on form!

PUNCH SIX
BALANCE

Working Balance

For so many reasons, "WORKING BALANCE" should have been one of the first things discussed in this manual. It is THAT important. Balance is the key to everything in your exercise routine, day to day living, and how you function safely and efficiently. There are many reasons for poor balance, from inner ear disturbances, poor nutrition, allergies, and sleep deprivation to neurological and/or developmental conditions or previous injuries. An imbalance great adversely affect how you walk, step, lift, squat, well...how you move. Poor balance can translate to alignment issues with your physical being and decreased abilities. In short, balance is everything.

By working with the Pas Fitness system, your balance will improve as will your confidence. Yes, balance and confidence are very much connected in how you perform, how you act, react, and how you grow as an athlete. The athlete within must discover balance before moving to the next level.

As you have read, balance is extremely important with punching, kicking, how you stand, and how to engage different muscle groups. From the fitness perspective, balance never gets boring. There are so many ways to challenge ourselves with balance exercise. Whether you are an Olympic athlete, an elementary school kickball champion or someone overcoming an injury or developmental issue, you can ALWAYS improve your balance.

Why Balance Matters

What if you were told that your balance could save you money? Literally, millions and millions of people around the world are injured, even hospitalized, due to poor balance and people with special needs have even greater costs but if you can improve your balance, you can improve your chances of staying and remaining healthier. To repeat: Medical issues can be helped if those with special needs are healthier, stronger, and have greater core and stability.

So What is Core and Stability?

Is having good balance really that important?

YES!

Everyone needs good balance but some people have more difficulty with balance. When you suffer from imbalance, often times this means there is poor core and stability issues.

Most people think of the "abs" or abdominals as your core but the truth is, the core is your entire core, your being. Your core includes your stomach muscles (abdominals) but also the internal and external obliques, the transversus and rectus abdominus. But the fact is…the core muscle group includes ALL of the muscles connected to your torso that keep the body stable and balanced. This is your super highway, the core that keeps you upright, strong, stable.

Your Superhighway

Your superhighway core can be split into two types of muscles: Stabilizers and Movers

- ***Stabilizers***: These are the muscles that attach directly to the spine and support its movement.
- ***Movers:*** The muscles that support the stabilizer muscles and work with them to move your body.

KNOW THIS! Balance = Independence!

SPECIAL NEEDS FACTS:
WHO IS MOST AFFECTED BY POOR BALANCE?

Cerebral Palsy

Spastic Cerebral Palsy is the most common diagnosis. Sufferers often complain of very stiff muscles and movements that appear (and feel) jerky. Spasticity is a form of hypertonia, an increased muscled tone.

Dyskinetic Cerebral Palsy is separated further into two different groups: athetoid and dystonic. Athetoid cerebral palsy includes cases with involuntary movement, especially in the arms, legs and hands. Dystonia/Dystonic cerebral palsy encompasses cases that affect the trunk muscles more than the limbs and results in fixed, twisted posture.

Ataxic Cerebral Palsy affects coordinated movements. Balance and posture are involved. Walking gait is often very wide and sometimes irregular. Control of eye movements and depth perception can be impaired. Often, fine motor skills requiring coordination of the eyes and hands, such as writing, are difficult.

Hypertonic results in awkward movements. The muscle's resistance can be tight causing spasms, as well as poor balance with random contractions in the muscles at any given time.

Hypotonic results in ragdoll appearance due to limp muscles. The head may fall backwards or side to side, causing difficulty maintaining posture, standing or walking without assistance, respiratory problems, and increased chance of autism.

Down Syndrome

The most common musculoskeletal effects of Down syndrome include weak muscle tone (***hypotonia***) and ligaments that are too loose (ligament laxity).
Note: This group is often misunderstood as we now know there is not enough research into the

hypotonia of children with Down syndrome and how that changes as they get older.

Williams Syndrome

Young children with Williams syndrome often have low muscle tone and joint laxity. As the children get older, joint stiffness (contractures) may develop. Physical therapy is very helpful in improving muscle tone, strength and joint range of motion.

The Reality of Special Needs

Every person is different!
We can no more say that all people with cerebral palsy move the same any more than we say all tall red-heads move the same. We are each unique; we are each gifted and challenged in various ways. Understanding our weaknesses, however, can only make us stronger!

KNOW THIS: If you simply give up because it is too hard to move, too hard to stand, too hard to test your balance, your quality of life WILL worsen over time.

SENIOR FACTS:

By 2030, 72 million Americans will be over the age of 65. Of the 38 million people we have today who are over the age of 65, only 22 percent are active. This is the #1 group most likely to fall and wind up in the emergency room.

Falls are the leading cause of injury among Americans over age 65, according to the federal Centers for Disease Control and Prevention (CDC). Each year, nearly one-third of older adults experience a fall, and 20 to 30 percent of them wind up with moderate to severe injuries, ranging from broken teeth to broken hips. In 2005, the CDC reports, 1.8 million elderly patients were treated in emergency rooms for non-fatal falls and 15,800 died of their injuries.

Some 20 to 40 percent of those suffering a hip fracture will die within a year, researchers estimate, but even lesser injuries can precipitate a cascade of medical problems, including the onset of severe disability, the end of independent living and the beginning of round-the-clock care. This spiral is tragic for the elderly patient, devastating for the family and expensive for the federal Medicare program. In 2000, falls cost more than $19 billion overall, the CDC estimates, with $12 billion going to hospitalizations, $4 billion to emergency room visits and $3 billion to outpatient care. By the year 2020, The Centers for Medicare and Medicaid Services projects the annual price tag for care related to falls among seniors will more than double to $43.8 billion.

Beyond falls…neglect of scoliosis, bad knee, hip, ankle, back issues all adversely affect your musculoskeletal being. Everything is connected.

INJURIES ARE PREVENTABLE!

Balance and Proprioception

Proprioception means your body's ability to interpret and use information about your position in space. That is, it is a learned skill set to interpret where and how you are standing, how close you are to a chair, or how high a step might be. Through a complex system of environmental feedback, cues from the bottom of your feet, the relation of your inner ear to gravity, to what you see, your body understands how to activate and use different muscles and/or change positions in movement. Each time you stand, get up from a chair, or walk across a room, you are using these senses. It also uses all of these cues when you're riding a bike, strength training at the gym, and standing on your tiptoes to grab something from a high shelf.

But when the information received is too complex to translate, the system gets overwhelmed and you lose your balance. You can, however, train to have better balance!

KNOW THIS: The greatest athletes in the world train to gain (and maintain) better balance. You can, too.

So, how is your balance? Let's test it!

Close Your Eyes Test

Few people know what the word "proprioception" means but you experience it every day all day long. It is your body's ability to interpret and understand the world around it and thus knows how to gauge distances, heights, widths of things around you. Your proprioception helps maintain balance and prevent falls. But what happens if you close your eyes while standing? Do you lose that perception?

Standing with your hands on your hips, feet shoulder width apart, close your eyes. The moment you feel any imbalance, open your eyes. But can you stand there with your eyes closed for 10 to 20 seconds? If so, you have reasonably good balance.

Straight Line Test

Imagine you are trying to walk a straight line, placing one foot directly in front of the other – heel to toe, heel to toe. Can you do it?

Now try to stand on that same line, heel to toe, and close your eyes? Have someone stand right next to you just for safety. Can you do it? If you begin to wobble, open your eyes before you fall!

Uneven Surface Test

Not only is the world round, it is uneven! Every day we tread on uneven surfaces and our bodies (not just our ankles) are forced to make very fast adjustments. Often times, when we are unable to make those quick transitions, we fall.

Standing on a foam pad or similar base, stand shoulder width apart with your hands on your hips. Can you hold your balance? Can you feel the muscles moving and twitching in your ankles, calves, and legs? Always be sure to have someone or something near you to hold on to once you feel any imbalance. If you have good balance, you should be able to hold your position on the uneven surface for up to 20 seconds.

Wide Leg/Close Leg Base Test

It is natural to stand with your feet shoulder width apart. This is your natural standing (and walking) stance. But can you put your feet together, ankles touching, hands on hips and hold your position? Do you wobble or are you rock steady?

As soon as you are able to perform the close leg base test (and not until then), try this next test.

One Leg Test

Hands on hips and feet almost shoulder width apart, try raising one leg. Note: Make sure you have a solid base, like a heavy chair or a pole next to you, so you have something to grab a hold of if needed. Safety first always!

Start with just lifting your heel and leave the toes on the floor. If you can master this, next lift the entire leg until you raise your knee up toward your hips. However, if you feel wobbly only raising the heel, no need to go any further.

If you can raise a knee and hold it, how long? Can you hold it for 10 to 20 seconds? Now try the other leg. Be warned: You may find that you have much better balance on one side than the other.

KNOW THIS: If you stare at a single focal point, you will be able to hold better balance. This is an old martial arts and yoga trick. Find your focal point.

Muscles Worked While You Fight for Balance

Want to take a guess at how hard you are working when you struggle to find balance in various positions? Here are just some of the muscles you work while trying to find your balance:

- Erector spinae
- Internal and external oblique
- Gluteus medius and minimus
- Gluteus maximus
- Rectus abdominus
- External oblique
- Adductor longus and abductor longus
- Vastus intermedius, vastus lateralis and vastus medialis
- Semitendinosus
- Semimembranosus
- Gastrocnemius
- Soleus, peroneus longus, flexor digitorum longus, and extensor digitorum longus

In other words, when you are able to hold your balance on uneven terrain, standing with a wide or narrow stance, or on one leg, you are working your entire core, lower back, and legs. You are in control of YOU!

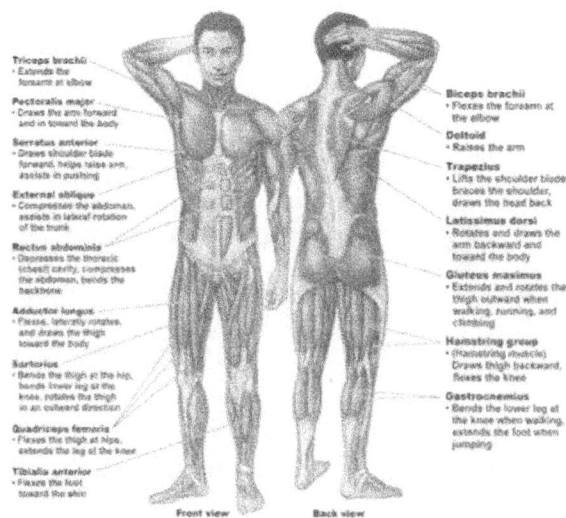

Take a moment to understand and appreciate how your body moves!

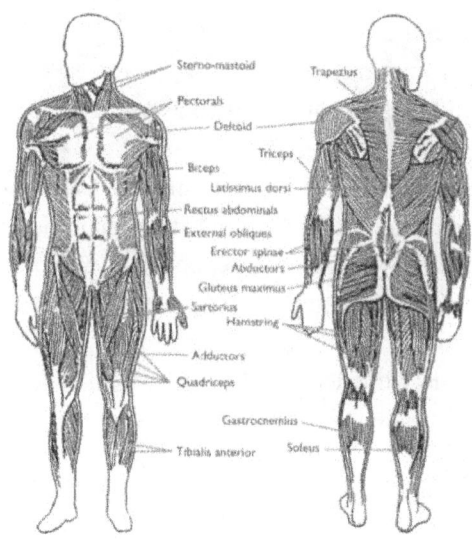

PUNCH SEVEN
I CAN'T HEAR YOU!

Your lungs are a muscle.

Did you know that?

Your lungs contain 1500 miles of airways and over 300 million alveoli. Every minute, you breathe 13 pints of air. Impressive.

Okay, but what happens when your air passage is diminished? For those who suffer with asthma, upper respiratory and/or bronchial issues, and for those with lung disease you already understand how precious breathing is. For most of us, however, we never really think about breathing. It's so easy, right?

But as we age, there is a natural atrophying (or weakening) of the muscles and nerve tissues that affect your vocal cords but you CAN train to have a stronger voice. Yes, you can. There is the belief that being vocally fit will allow you to have a stronger voice as you age. But who thinks about healthy voice exercises?

There are many things you can do to maintain stronger vocal chords. Read out loud for 10 to 15 minutes two or three times a week. Sing along with the radio or join a choir. If you take a fitness class, count along with the instructors while you perform repetitions. As an instructor, I can promise you that we (instructors) love it when our classes count along! As you exercise, learning to speak is an invaluable tool. You are learning to control your breathing, your diaphragm, and measure how you take in and expel oxygen. Talking or counting out loud while exercising is a skill all to itself.

This is why we yell in martial arts.

Pas Fitness

In martial arts, there are different kinds of art forms and what we call "the yell." It is called the "kia" or the "kihai" or "hi-ya!" In tae kwon do, a Korean form of martial arts, it is the "k'ihap." Whatever your preference, there is a reason for the yell.

    1. Increased power!
    2. It sounds cool!

3. You mean business!

KNOW THIS: When you can "yell," you have better posture!

Each time you yell as you are about to strike, you tighten your abdominal muscles and flex those vocal chords! You are working your core to project power. It ensures that you breathe out (exhale) at the proper time and you learn how to breathe better.

Each time you yell as you are about to strike, it creates better form and technique. You are not throwing a random punch or aimlessly kicking but you are projecting precision and power, thought and effort!

Each time you yell as you are about to strike, you gain more confidence in your movement. You are literally training your entire body to move on instinct, to project power, better and safer movements, and are ingraining certain movements to muscle memory.

What is Muscle Memory?

It was once believed that once a person stopped working out or stopped using certain muscles due to injury or illness, those once tuned muscles were lost forever. What we know now, however, is that when movements are repeated over time, long-term memory in the body, in the muscles, is established. It is engrained in your body and mind so that you can perform a task, such as opening a lock, typing, or riding a bike, without conscious effort.

Muscle Memory, Pas Fitness and Special Needs

In a new study looking at toddlers and preschoolers with autism, researchers found that children with better motor skills were more adept at socializing and communicating.[12] And, in fact, this study supports a growing number of different studies linking motor skills and muscle memory to better health, better balance, better welfare to those with Down syndrome and cerebral palsy.[13]

Muscle Memory, Pas Fitness and Parkinson's Disease

Parkinson's disease is a debilitating, neurodegenerative disease that can be fast-acting and devastating to one's muscle, coordination, and mobility. As the disease progresses, quality of life can be diminished but more studies have found that exercises that promote cognitive skills, balance and posture drills, repetition, and power can restore muscle and better movement.[14]

---

[12] https://www.psychologytoday.com/blog/the-athletes-way/201309/how-is-the-cerebellum-linked-autism-spectrum-disorders
[13] http://www.newswise.com/articles/non-traditional-therapy-for-kids-with-cerebral-palsy-shows-effective
[14] https://www.uab.edu/medicine/news/latest/item/329-strength-training-shows-benefit-for-parkinson-s-patients

For Parkinson's patients, aerobic exercises that improve mobility, posture, balance, and gait, in addition to learning-based memory exercises (engaging muscle memory) can be lifesaving.[15]

What's more, exercising the vocal cords is critically important for those with Parkinson's disease.

KNOW THIS: Not only are we capable of great things, but we're capable of rewiring our own brains and muscles. It just takes practice. A lot of practice.

So…How DO You Yell?

In Pas Fitness, we ask that you deliver quick, loud K'ihap or Hi-ya's but the noise should be clipped. "Hiy'" or "Ki" or "Hey" so that every yell, every noise is forced from the diaphragm with power.

As you punch – "Hiy!"
As you kick – "Ki!"

It requires that you expel air while you explode with a powerful punch or kick. You are breathing! You are tightening the abdominals. You are strong!

(Note: Watch our videos to see how to yell and execute power.)

---

[15] http://pdcenter.neurology.ucsf.edu/patients-guide/exercise-and-physical-therapy

PUNCH EIGHT
HOW TO MOVE!

I was working with trainer Micah Stewart the first time I heard the reference of working with good neighbors. I looked around. Who was he talking about? As it happened, he was talking about my knee.

I've had three knee surgeries, two broken ankles, a plethora of back and hip flexor issues, and all before the age of 30. Today, decades later, I am stronger and healthier than I have ever been. I have good neighbors.

But even now, if I am tired or not paying attention, it is easy for me to compensate my body's position, placing more weight on my right leg/knee in an effort to spare my left (worst) knee.

Every day in gyms everywhere, trainers see this very subtle, very slight movement that no one else notices. A person with a bad back leans to one side, perhaps shifting a hip to the side. Another person with a bad knee unconsciously shifts weight to the other leg with every squat or lunge. Yet another jeopardizes proper posture of the back in order to compensate for a bad shoulder. These are just a few examples of how people make seemingly minor body adjustments that can cause more harm than good to the body while working out. How you move has direct impact on how strong you can become and how efficiently you can move.

KNOW THIS: As you get better mobility, better stability, and better balance, this makes a HUGE impact on your functional movement, which enables better neighbors.

So, what is a Good Neighbor?

In physical therapy it is very common to see a patient with a knee pain that is caused by a hip injury or hip pain cause by a bad back. Many times pain in an ankle, knee, hip, back, elbow, wrist or shoulder is being caused by an entirely different body part. That "bad" neighbor (the actual muscle or joint that is weak or injured) can wreak havoc all over your body. In your quest to have good neighbors, you must determine if and where your bad neighbors are!

Now that you understand how important balance and stability are, you can see why and how core and stability training is so important to having a strong, healthy body. When you practice Pas Fitness, you are creating a strong new you.

As you train and exercise, pay attention to your body. Note the improvements you make in your balance, posture, coordination, strength and agility!

You ARE an athlete!
You CAN do this!

Okay, here comes to the good stuff. In the next few pages, we will begin to truly understand the importance of core and stability. In Chapter (Punch) One, the issue of money was introduced. Poor health, instability, and weak muscles cost you money.

Fitness Saves Money!

A beautiful example of this was documented by a fire academy instructor, Captain Contreras, when he began to learn more about functional movement and what it is. Captain Contreras was introduced to a relatively new program called Functional Movement Systems (FMS) and became curious how this system could decrease the number of injuries he saw with his fire fighters. What he was interested in was not only protecting his personnel but also saving money on medical and insurance costs.

What is FMS and Why Should We Care?

The concept is brilliant. Simply, it is a screening that tests seven different movement patters (visit www.functionalmovement.com)and offers scores on each test and movement. The test must be conducted by a certified FMS instructor. The scoring scale is:

- 0 – Participant receives a 0 if there is pain connected to the movement. The participant should be referred to a healthcare professional.
- 1 – Participant is unable to perform or complete a functional movement pattern.
- 2 – Participant is able to perform the functional pattern but with some degree of compensation.
- 3 – Participant was able to easily/efficiently perform the functional movement pattern.

A 21 is considered to be the perfect or ideal score for functional movement.

When Contreras put his recruits through the FMS program, he learned that those who received a total of 14 points or less were three times more likely to become injured. In fact, he discovered that those who scored a 14 or lower were also identified to have decreased work capacity compared to those recruits who tested with a 15 or higher in their FMS assessment.

Following the academy, all recruits were then monitored within the system for two to three-and-a-half years, depending on when they had completed their training. Fourteen recruits were broken into two groups: those who scored 14 and below and those who scored 15 and above. When Contreras broke the recruits into two groups, he found that the expenditures of worker's compensation were six times more for the 14 and under group and overall costs to those injured were higher with the 14 and under group. Bottom line: Those with better movement were less likely to be injured and when they were, the injures were (overall) less significant and less expensive.

In yet another report, very similar findings resulted with FMS tests within the NFL. What is so interesting is that fire fighters and professional football players are, as a whole, a strong, young, athletic group of people and yet look how many struggle with proper movement, balance, agility, stability and ability.[16]

Pas Fitness has created its own B.A.S.I.C.S. program which is a series of assessment tests for those with special needs to determine where your strengths and weaknesses may lie in gross motor skills, balance, cognitive thinking, functional movement, and confidence! (check out References for more information).

Whether you are an Olympic athlete, a senior citizen, a person with a physical disability, or just someone who wants to get into better physical condition, you can learn to move more efficiently and feel stronger than ever before!

KNOW THIS: The "practice makes perfect" is truer than you can image. Practice reduces injury, practice instills confidence but it must be a good practice. If you practice bad form, it is more than an imperfect practice…it could be an unhealthy one.

So, How Do I Move Properly?
"Put Your Back into It!"

No! Please don't!

Let's just take the common everyday (in the gym) leg stretch. As people begin to stretch, they reach for the toes and the back rolls out. People are so focused on reaching their toes, they can do more harm to the back.

What is one of the number one things that sends people to the emergency room on Thanksgiving morning? The turkey. No, not from overeating. In fact, it most often happens before the turkey is even cooked. With heavy bird in hand, proper form is forgotten.

As strong and marvelous as the human body is, the back (spinal column) is very susceptible to injury. A weaker core allows your back to roll outward putting undue (and very unhealthy) stress on the back.

KNOW THIS: Your lower back should be flat or even slightly concaved (as though there is a slight arch in the back) with your core engaged!

Gorilla vs. Chicken

---

[16] https://experiencelife.com/article/fms-screen-test

Which would you like to be?

You would probably guess the gorilla and…you would be wrong. Gorillas look strong and sound ferocious. Were we to swing from the jungle vines and wildly beat our chests, the whole gorilla thing could work. But if we're talking about grocery shopping, simply doing everyday activities, or just walking, you really do want to be a chicken. With our long and vulnerable spinal cord, we really want to walk like a chicken.

While the gorilla is slumped forward, shoulders rolled forward, the back is terribly out of alignment, the chicken has got it going on!

Chest up, shoulder blades (or chicken wings) pulled together, and chin up, everything is in alignment. Your head is set back so that your ears are over your shoulder and the shoulders are even with your hips and hips are aligned with your ankles. In this position, everything is set to protect the back.

KNOW THIS: The average adult head weighs between 10 to 12 pounds, already putting a strain on the body if one does not have proper body posture.

It can be the most seemingly innocent things, like texting or putting a turkey in the oven that hurt you simply because your body is in poor alignment.

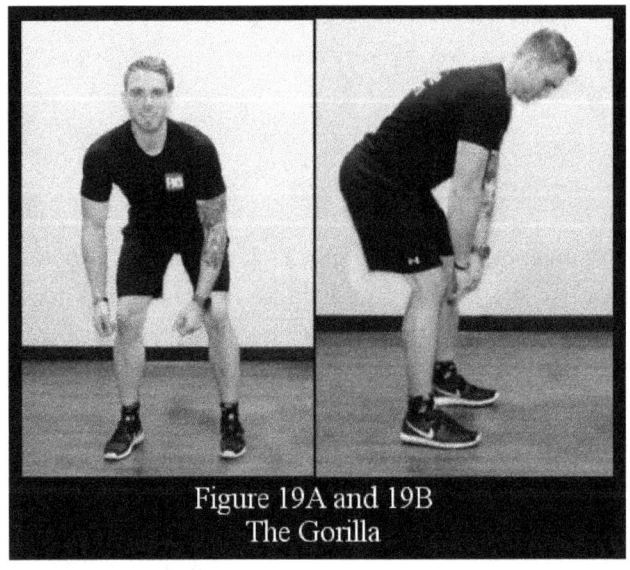

Figure 19A and 19B
The Gorilla

Note how his back is rolled out, leaving his spine unprotected.

Walk Like a Chicken, Feel Like a Gorilla

Okay, so maybe you don't want to walk around the grocery store like a chicken, but you can come close. And who ever saw a chicken with a bad back? As mentioned before, how you move directly impacts your back.

- Pull back your shoulder blades or engage scapular retraction.
- Lift your chin up.
- Engage your core. Imagine you could be punched in the stomach and hold your abdominal muscles while still breathing. Hold…hold…hold.
- Tilt your pelvis slightly, straightening the lower back and engaging the lower back muscles or spinal erectae.
- Do the chicken check: Are your ears over your shoulder? Your shoulders over your hips? Your hips over your ankles?

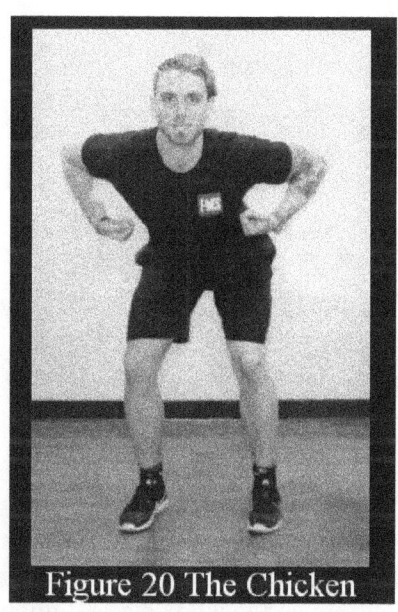

Figure 20 The Chicken

Chickens Don't Text

Studies support that over 80 percent of Americans between the ages of 14 to 44 have their cell phones with them up to 22 hours each day. Cell phone users between the ages of 18 and 24 send upward to 70 texts per day, and teenagers send approximately 100 texts, according to a 2013 study by the Pew Research Center. Add to this Instagram, SnapChat, Facebook, Twitter, and other social media sites and/or electronic devices that have the user looking down. In a new study by the Journal of Behavioral Addictions, women spend an average of 10 hours a day on cell phones. Forgoing concerns about relationships, work, and productivity habits, what is this doing to our physical well-being?

What Happens When You Text?

Without even thinking about it, you assume a position when you text. You've seen others doing it a hundred times. The head drops down, the shoulders pinch and roll forward, and suddenly there is an instant slump in the back. Over time, these stresses could lead to wear and tear, degeneration of the spine, and possible surgeries.

Standing upright, with shoulders back, abdominal muscles engaged, ears over (in line with) shoulders, there is zero pressure on the spine. However, as soon as you look down toward the cell phone, gravity takes over. The following is just how much damage is being done the more and the further your head drops down.

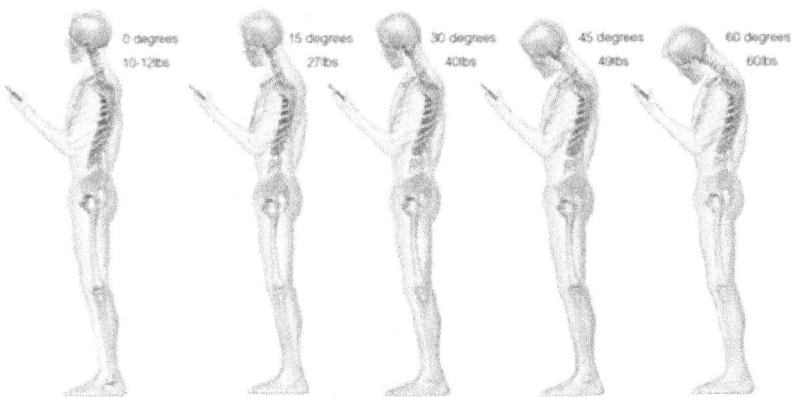

- At a 15-degree bend of the neck, the weight of your head feels like 27 pounds.
- At a 30-degree bend of the neck, the weight of your head feels like 40 pounds.
- At a 45-degree bend of the neck, the weight of your head feels like 49 pounds.
- At a 60-degree bend of the neck, the weight of your head feels like 60 pounds.

What Else Can Chickens Do?
  ... why, they can squat!

In my Silver Sneaker classes, my spin and kickbox classes, my bootcamps, Pilates, even martial arts classes, perhaps the most "I can't do" I hear for a requested task is the squat.

But a squat is real life. When you drop something and need to bend down to retrieve it, when you have to step into a low riding car or need to get up for a low seat, these are real life activities that require a squat and yet so many people insist they cannot do it.

I SAY SQUAT, YOU SAY...
"It's bad for my knees."
"I can't squat."
"Squatting hurts my knees!"

The Myth About Squats

Squatting is one of the most basic movements in human life. Every day you emulate "the squat" each time you get in and out of your car, sit or stand, bend to pick something up, and even get into bed. This body function is an undeniable part of our lives yet we believe that we should not perform the task as it might hurt or cause more damage to our knees and back.

The Truth About Squats

If you are mobile, if you are a senior, if you do hope to stay active and want a better quality of life, you WANT to squat! In fact, squatting is actually good for your knees. Squats offer you more flexibility in the hips and strength in the legs allows you to step higher. Stepping up into your car, bathtub, up on a curb, climbing stairs and even negotiating uneven surfaces, the additional flexibility will help avoid stumbling and falling.

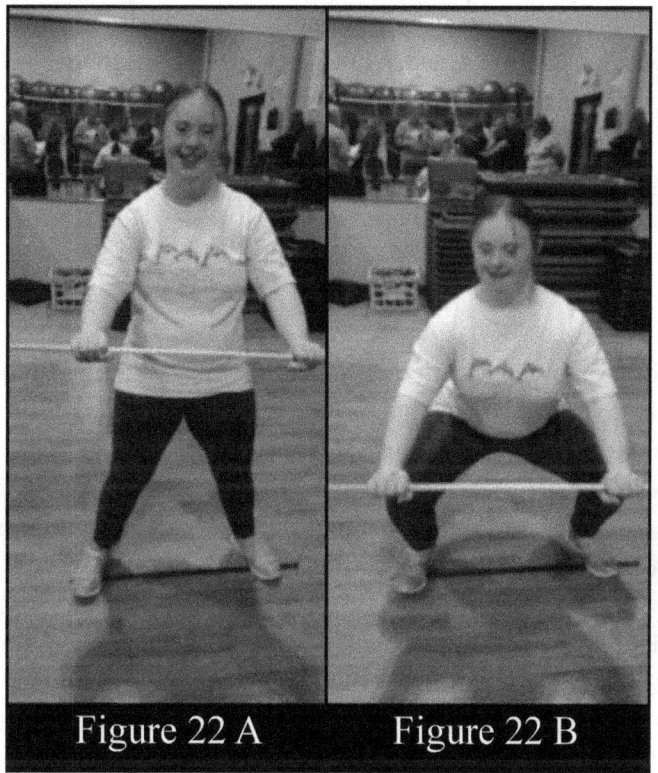

Figure 22 A   Figure 22 B

Squat = Independence

Jamie is lined up perfectly on a line and using a dowel to keep her shoulders and hands level and steady. Next, in Figure 25b, (while smiling!) Jamie executes a perfect squat!

Squat to Live...And Live to Squat

- When you squat, you build better muscles (including a stronger back, quadriceps, hamstrings, glutes and calves), but it also helps improve overall muscle mass in the body. Loss of muscle is a battle every senior must be ready to fight!
- When you squat, it allows you to continue those real-life activities such as retrieving groceries from the car, picking up a grandchild, even picking up the morning paper.

- When you squat, it increases balance, stabilizing muscles and becoming far more centered. With a squat comes greater leg strength and more stability. Squats also strengthen the inner thighs, which weaken as we age.
- When you squat, you build stronger muscles, ligaments, and connective tissues. All of this enables you to better prevent injuries.
- When you squat, you burn more fat.
- When you squat, you build stronger ankles.
- When you squat, you build stronger knees.
- When you squat, you build a stronger back and hips.
- When you squat, you help protect your body against obesity, diabetes, and cardiovascular disease. Greater muscle and muscle ignition helps the body to regulate glucose, lipid metabolism and insulin sensitivity in the body.
- When you squat, it actually improves the manner in which your body handles fluids, delivering nutrients to organs and muscle tissue but also through the colon, allowing for more regular bowel movements.

How to Squat

Even if you feel too weak in the legs to do a squat properly, you can improve! For beginners, squat from your bed rather than a chair or use a chair with armrests and push against the rests to stand. Over time, you can move from the bed or use the armrests less and less.

Go for the assisted squat! Hold onto something solid to keep from falling backwards. This is important. Most people lean forward in the squat and this puts more strain on both the back and knees. But a proper squat will actually improve knee stability and connective tissue.

1. Stand with your feet just over shoulder width apart and toes out 15 degrees.
2. Keep looking forward. Do not drop your head forward or your chin down.
3. Keep your back in a neutral position and keep your knees centered over your feet.
4. Slowly bend your knees, hips, and ankles, lowering until you reach a 90-degree angle. Imagine your bottom is dropping down toward your heels. Make sure feet are flat.
5. Return to starting position, using your legs and hips to return to the standing position. Drive up, pushing on the heels. Note: If you used more arm strength (or pull) than leg/hip push, you must continue to work on leg strength.
6. Breathe in as you lower, breathe out as you return to the starting position. Repeat 15-20 times, for 2-3 sets for beginners. Do this two or three times a week.

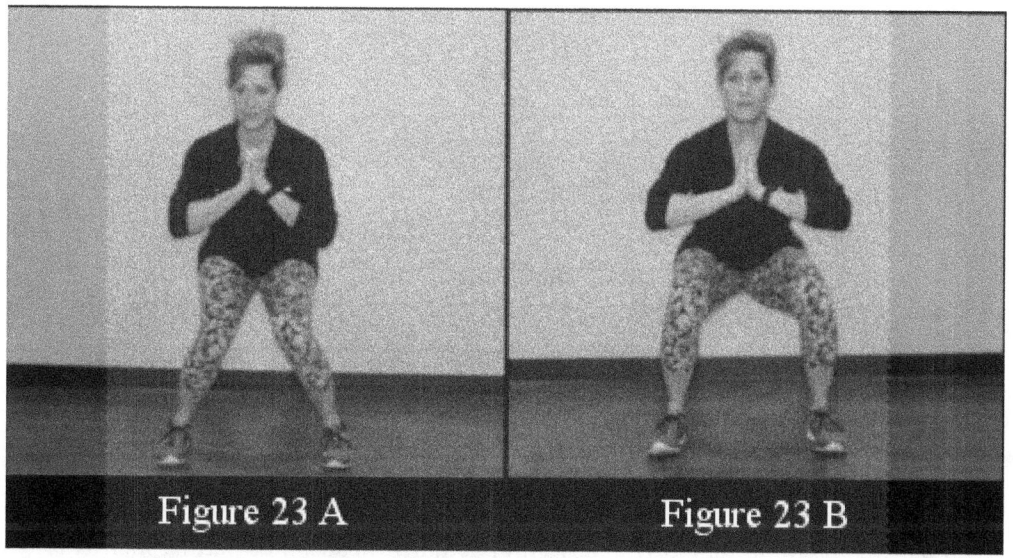

In Figure 23A, notice how Dionne is folding inward and her knees are collapsing in. In Figure 23B, she is strong. Her head is up, back straight, knees forward.

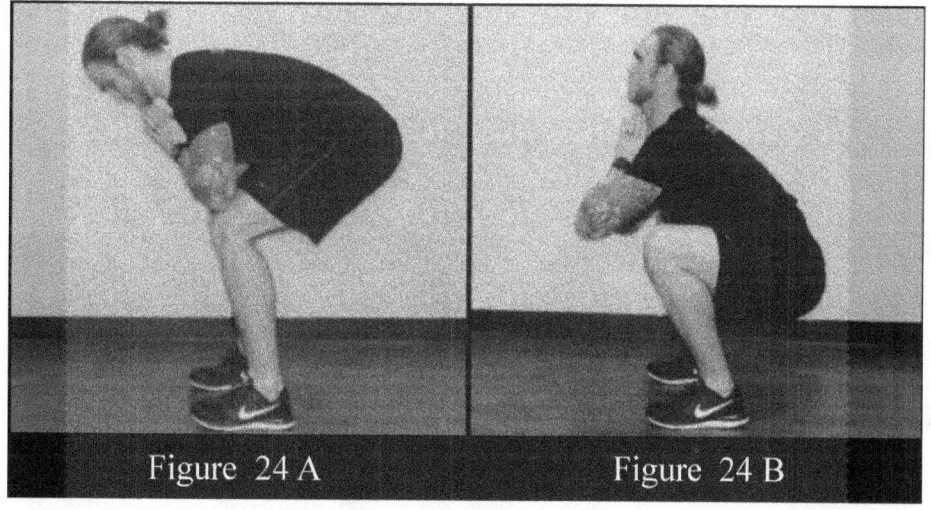

Figure 24A depicts one of the most common mistakes we see when asking a person to perform a squat. As he looks downward, his body tips forward. Movement is limited.

In Figure 27B, Micah is performing the perfect squat.

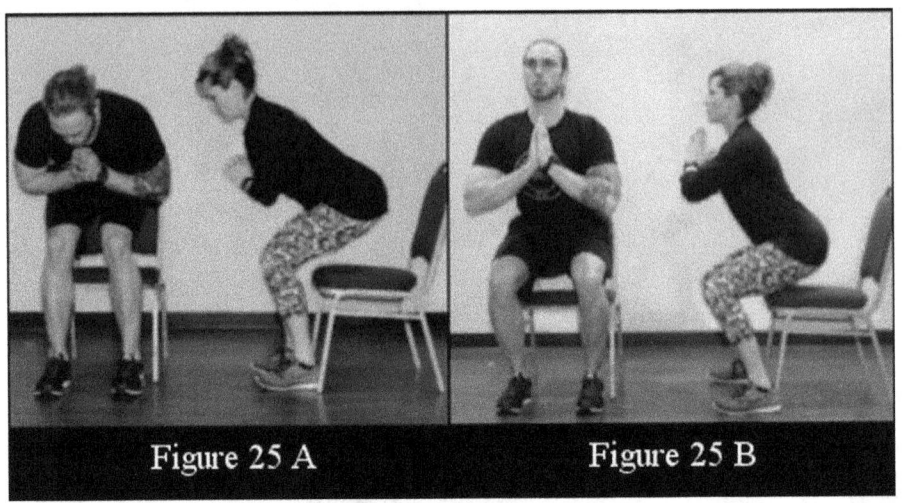

Figure 25 A   Figure 25 B

In Figure 25A, both Dionne and Micah have dropped their heads, thus putting their backs and bodies out of alignment with a strong squat. Micah's back is rolled out while Dionne's knees are caving inward.

But in Figure 25B, both Dionne and Micah have perfect posture and are protecting their backs, knees, and hips while performing a good squat.

In this chapter, you learned to be aware of your own body, your posture, how you carry yourself, and how proper body alignment can prevent injuries and make you stronger!

The final informational chapter is perhaps the most exciting as you will learn how to put everything together. This is your guide to improving your life.

PUNCH NINE
THIS MOVES FOR YOU ... PAS FITNESS

Before beginning any exercise regimen, you know you must get permission from your personal physician. Every person and body is different so please speak to your physician, show him or her this manual, and be sure that you may perform these exercises. As a general rule, people are so much stronger than they think they are but without knowing your personal medical history, it is unsafe to encourage you to do something that may not be beneficial.

Got a green light from your doctor? Then let's do this! In the Pas Fitness exercises, you will develop all the things we have discussed to become stronger and healthier. In addition to the punches and kicks, here is what you are going to learn:

Top Ten Power Moves to Make You Stronger as You Punch and Kick!

1. Balance Holds. These involve single leg stands, knee raises and leg swings.
2. Squats. This includes assisted squats and chair squats.
3. One-legged exercises to develop core strength, balance, and independence!
4. Heel Raises
5. Push-Ups or Push-Ups on the wall
6. Cross Patterns
7. Crossing the Line leg work for better balance
8. Abdominals
9. Superman
10 .Bridges

Whether you are 15 or 75 years old, these are all exercises you want to be able to perform for real life situations. If you fall down, you want to be able to pull yourself up or certainly at least pull yourself to safety. You want to restore coordination, be strong, and have good energy to enjoy life. These are all the exercises that will best help you find that happier and healthier you.

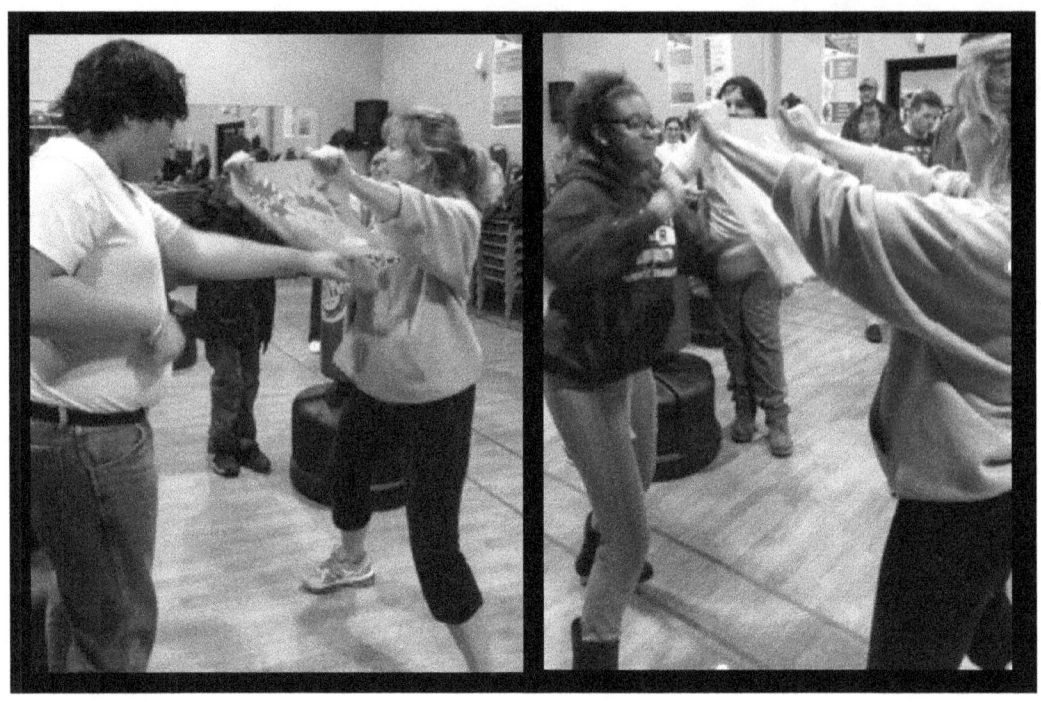

PUNCH TEN
YOUR INTRODUCTION TO PAS FITNESS AND EMPOWERMENT!

This is it. You have seen all the pictures throughout the book of people smiling and laughing while punching on the target paper. Here is your introduction to Pas Fitness and your moment of truth!!

Take a moment and look at the pictures again.

When students of Pas Fitness are punching, they are learning to stabilize their core. Imagine, for example, the importance of being able to lean over a sink to brush your teeth without assistance or having to lean against the counter for support. Most people do not even think about this act as being "able-bodied" but it is. The physical act of being able to stand, lean forward, then stand straight again is one of independence, stability and strength. Punching helps to gain this independence.

When students of Pas Fitness are punching, they are learning to maintain balance. Each time the hands extend forward, away from the body, the very weight of your arms suddenly challenge your core strength and balance. As you punch, your abdominal, back, shoulders, even leg muscles are all engaged to maintain balance as you strike the target. This is huge! So many muscles are in play.

Before you try the workout programs offered later in the book, start with punching.

Simple punches.

As instructed earlier (and if you have forgotten, return to Punch Five: Getting Started and look at the "How to Punch" section), you are going to punch.

<u>Here's what you need:</u>
A Pas Fitness target
A partner

Gloves (optional)

KNOW THIS: You can save money on gloves and try this -- put socks on your hands to protect your skin from the target material and punch. As long as your thumb is on the OUTSIDE of your fist as you punch and not tucked inside the fist, socks make a great alternative to more expensive gloves.

See the FOUR CIRCLES on your target paper? Have your partner call out to which circles to punch on.

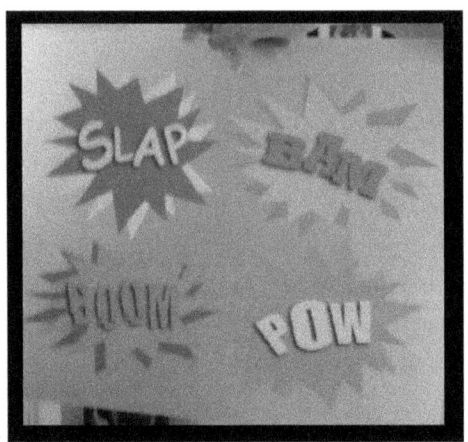

Example: This target has words but you can get a target sheet with 1, 2, 3, and 4, or even colors.

Pas Fitness will let you pick your own words, letters, colors or numbers. Go for it.

Partner 1:
1-2-1-2 punches = 20 seconds
Left side forward
Left punch – circles 1 & 3 = 20 seconds
Right side forward
Right punch – circles 2 & 4 = 20 seconds
1-2-1-2 punches = 20 seconds
Left side forward
Left punch – circles 1 & 4 = 20 seconds
Right side forward
Right punch – circles 2 & 3 = 20 seconds

Partner 2:
1-2-1-2 punches = 20 seconds
Left side forward
Left punch – circles 1 & 3 = 20 seconds
Right side forward
Right punch – circles 2 & 4 = 20 seconds
1-2-1-2 punches = 20 seconds
Left side forward
Left punch – circles 1 & 4 = 20 seconds
Right side forward
Right punch – circles 2 & 3 = 20 seconds

That was TWO MINUTES of punching! Ready for more?

If and when you are ready for more ….

Partner 1:
1-2-1-2 punches = 20 seconds
Left side = 20 seconds
Right side = 20 seconds
1-2-1-2 punches = 30 seconds
Left side = 30 seconds
Right side = 30 seconds
1-2-1-2 punches = 40 seconds
Left side = 40 seconds
Right side = 40 seconds
1-2-1-2 punches = 50 seconds
Left side = 50 seconds
Right side = 50 seconds

Partner 2:
1-2-1-2 punches = 20 seconds
Left side = 20 seconds
Right side = 20 seconds
1-2-1-2 punches = 30 seconds
Left side = 30 seconds
Right side = 30 seconds
1-2-1-2 punches = 40 seconds
Left side = 40 seconds
Right side = 40 seconds

1-2-1-2 punches = 50 seconds
Left side = 50 seconds
Right side = 50 seconds

Wow!

Get creative! Each time you cross jab, call out new circles to punch, you are not only working your core and muscles but you are also having to recall patterns and exercising your brain as well. This is a fantastic workout for everyone!

PAS FITNESS
TARGET TRAINING
PHASE I

In Pas Fitness training, we want to work balance, ability, stability, better movement, better posture and confidence! To do all these great things, it is always wise to keep your routine fun and challenging. There are THREE workouts provided for you:

- Pas Fitness Target – Duration: 2-3 times per week
- Pas Fitness Circuit – Duration: 1 time per week
- Pas Fitness Stability – Duration: 1-2 times per week

You will need your Pas Fitness target, water and a great attitude! You can do this! Make sure you have room to move!

Warm-up (three to five minutes)

- Jabs
- Squats with jabs
- Invisible punching bag

  - Those squats with the jabs can be very small if needed. If you cannot squat well, just make small squat motions – always be comfortable. You can do this!
  - If you are seated, attempt to raise alternate legs (even just a half inch if that is what you can do) with each punch.

Here we go ….

With the Pas Fitness target in front of you, turn sideways. We are starting on your left side so put your left foot forward. Draw up your fists and let's go…

Cardio

The Jab

- Front jab (working the left side first)
- Front jab (right side)
- Front jab (left side)
- Front jab (right side)
- Front jab (left side)
- Front jab (right side)
   = Count of 16 on each side, every set!

- Front jab/back jab (working the left side first)
- Front jab/back jab (right side)
- Front jab/back jab (left side)
- Front jab/back jab (right side)
   = Count of 16 on each side, every set!

**AND REMEMBER WHAT WE TALKED ABOUT?
YELL LOUDLY AS YOU COUNT
…and don't forget to breathe!**

1-2-1-2 Punches

Facing the Pas Fitness target as though you are sitting on a horse:

- Punching 1-2-1-2 with strong and long punches.
(Forgot how to do this? Check out 1-2-1-2 Punches in the manual.)
   = 30 seconds
- Punching 1-2-1-2 with strong and long punches.
   = 30 seconds
- Punching 1-2-1-2 with strong and long punches.
   = 30 seconds

The Jab and The Hook

Turn to the side again, starting with your left side. We are going to combine the jab and a hook punch:

- Front jab/front hook (left side)

- Front jab/front hook (right side)
- Front jab/front hook (left side)
- Front jab/front hook (right side)
    = Count of 16 on each side, every rep.

KEEP COUNTING LOUDLY!
…and remember that if you cannot do it all, that is OKAY!
Use the chart to fill in the numbers you CAN do and be determined to do just one more punch the next time. This is all about becoming stronger. You can do this!

The Upper Cut

Adjust the Pas Fitness target so that it is lying flat. It is time for upper cuts! Alternating upper cuts so that you perform a left upper cut and then a right upper cut, back to the left upper cut, then the right upper cut…and so on. Count each upper cut. Once again, you are positioned as though you are sitting on a horse.

- Upper cuts
    = 30 seconds
- Upper cuts
    = 30 seconds
- Upper cuts
    = 30 seconds

Adding Kicks

- If you cannot kick, focus on just trying to lift your leg with this move. This helps to strengthen hip flexors, quads, glutes, as well as balance, your core and stability! So, give it a try.
- If you are seated, the same rules apply. If you can, attempt to raise that leg.

Front Kick

Turn the Pas Fitness target so that it is lying flat. Steady your balance. Remember to raise the knee first before kicking:

- Front kick (left side)
- Front kick (right side)
- Front kick (left side)
- Front kick (right side)
- Front kick (left side)
- Front kick (right side)

= Count of 16

Round Kick

Standing sideways, draw your fists up toward your chin and kick out to the side. Remember, form is very important. You are working balance and core!

- Round kick (left side)
- Round kick (right side)
- Round kick (left side)
- Round kick (right side)
- Round kick (left side)
- Round kick (right side)

= Count of 16

Front Kick with a Knee Up

After each front kick, return foot to the floor and quickly bring up the knee, return to floor and repeat. Kick. Knee up. Kick. Knee up. Note: A front kick and a knee up counts as ONE.

- Front kick/knee up (left side)
- Front kick/knee up (right side)
- Front kick/knee up (left side)
- Front kick/knee up (right side)
- Front kick/knee up (left side)
- Front kick/knee up (right side)

= Count of 16

1-2-1-2 Punches

Facing the Pas Fitness target as though you are sitting on a horse:

- Punching 1-2-1-2 with strong and long punches.
  = 30 seconds
- Punching 1-2-1-2 with strong and long punches.
  = 30 seconds
- Punching 1-2-1-2 with strong and long punches.
  = 30 seconds

Modified Crescent Kick

Because the crescent kick is an advanced kick, we need to modify the movement. When the knee is bent, this is a great flexion movement for the hips. It works balance, ability and agility but it IS CHALLENGING! Make sure you are stable enough to do this. Safety is always first.

Facing the Pas Fitness target, bend the knee as you raise the leg and make and outward sweeping motion with the leg, leading with the knee. Imagine that your knee is going to strike the target.

- Outside crescent knee-up (left side)
- Outside crescent knee-up (right side)
- Outside crescent knee-up (left side)
- Outside crescent knee-up (right side)
- Outside crescent knee-up (left side)
- Outside crescent knee-up (right side)

= Count of 12

Combination – Outside Crescent Knee-Up with Double Hooks

Let's bring in a combination. This is far more challenging so if you have to slow it down, take your time. Remember to have good form. Stand tall. Breathe.

As soon as you perform the crescent kick/knee-up, set the foot down and throw a (same side as the active leg) hook punch and then the back hook punch. Repeat.

- Outside crescent knee-up with left hook/right hook combination (left side)
- Outside crescent knee-up with right hook/left hook combination (right side)
- Outside crescent knee-up with left hook/right hook combination (left side)
- Outside crescent knee-up with right hook/left hook combination (right side)
- Outside crescent knee-up with left hook/right hook combination (left side)
- Outside crescent knee-up with right hook/left hook combination (right side)

= Count of 12

Cool Down

Nice job!!

Take down the intensity with some light punches again and add some bob and weave movement. Let your breathing return to normal.

Are you hot and sweaty? Good job!

In the chapter on balance (Punch Six), all the muscles utilized while performing balance holds was listed and it was pretty impressive. You just worked all those muscles and much, much more. With the added punches, hooks and upper cuts, you also worked:

- Trapezius

- Teres minor
- Teres major
- Pectoralis major
- Deltoid
- Biceps brachi
- Triceps brachi
- Serratus anterior
- As well as the abdominal and low back muscles listed with those balance holds.

Again – wow! Nice job. You have worked everything.

After a minute or two of light punches with a bob and weave, let's stretch.

Shoulder Shrugs

Pinch up the shoulders and hold for five seconds. Release and exhale. Ahhh! Repeat.
= 5 times

Shoulder Shrugs – rolling forward

Roll your shoulders forward with big circles but keep your back straight, head held high.
= 5 times

Shoulder Shrugs – rolling backwards

Roll your shoulders backwards, also in big circles. Chin up, back straight.
= 5 times

Straight Arm Stretch

Extend your right arm out in front of you. Place your left hand behind your right elbow and gently pull the arm in toward you. This should feel good. Do not continue to pull inward if this does not feel good.
Release.
Stretch the other side.
= hold each stretch for a good 10-20 seconds

Leg Stretch

On this stretch, posture is everything! Do NOT be a gorilla! No rolled backs. So…whether you are standing or seated, pull your toes back toward your knee. Straighten your back. Do NOT reach for your toes. Everyone always reaches for the toes. It is unnecessary and also causes you to roll the back! Lift your chin and imagine you are directing everything toward the knees. Toes and chins are pulled to the knee. Feel that? Oh, yes! That is an excellent stretch that you will feel from your mid-calf all the way up the leg.

Again – this is supposed to feel good.

Be A Chicken

Oh, the glorious chicken!

It is time to be nice to your back, to your knees, to your hips, and to your shoulders so let's be a chicken.

Head up, chin up.

Pull your shoulders back. Chest up. Create a nice straight (and strong) line for your back.

Now bend your knees very slightly and poke your bottom out just a little.

Can you imagine how a chicken walks?

Stand up and try that again!
And again!

Let's Go Bowling

Let's start with the right side.

Imagine you have a bowling ball in your hand. Bring it up toward you chin, then pull the imaginary ball back as your opposite leg (left) steps forward. Gently swing your bowling ball arm forward while performing a slight forward lunge. Nice job.

Are you watching your back?

Just as if you were really bowling, make sure your back is strong, abdominal muscles are tightened, chin is up, shoulders and back are NOT rounded.

= Bowl 3 strikes!

Let's move to the left side.

The ball is in your left hand so as you draw the imaginary ball back, step forward with your right leg. Slight lunge. Chin up, back straight and abs strong.

= Bowl 3 strikes!

Let's Play Some Ball

You did a lot of punching and hooks so let's make sure your back and shoulders are nice and loose. Imagine you are playing basketball. Dribble your imaginary ball three times then take a shot. Let your hand stay up in the air for a moment (just like the pro NBA stars!) and repeat.

= Take 3 shots!

Repeat on other side.   = Take 3 shots!

KNOW THIS: This was a big workout and you used all your muscles. If you cannot complete the entire workout that is OKAY! I tell all my classes, from beginners to the very advanced, from college students to senior citizens, the goal to working out is to grow, get stronger, and feel good. Do what you can, mark down your successes. By marking down what you can do, you will also be able to see your own personal growth. Perhaps today you are only able to do half (or less) than the workout. That is okay! But write down what you did and stick with it. Soon enough, you will get stronger. You will punch and kick harder. You will punch and kick faster. You will have better balance. Go for it!

Most people quit before they get the full benefit of a great workout.
Don't cheat yourself!

The Pas Fitness Target Workout

Punches				
Jab-left side				
Jab-right side				
Jab/Back Jab-left side				
Jab/Back Jab-right side				
1-2-1-2 Punches (30 seconds each)				
Jab/Hook-left side				
Jab/Hook-right side				
Upper Cuts (30 seconds each)				

Kicks				
Front Kick-left side				
Front Kick-right side				
Round House-left side				
Round House-right side				

Kicks & Punches				
Front Kick/Knee Up-left side				
Front Kick/Knee Up-right side				
1-2-1-2 Punches (30 seconds each)				
Outside Crescent Knee-Up-left				
Outside Crescent Knee-Up-right				
Outside Crescent w/Hooks-left				
Outside Crescent w/Hooks-right				
Cool Down/Stretch				

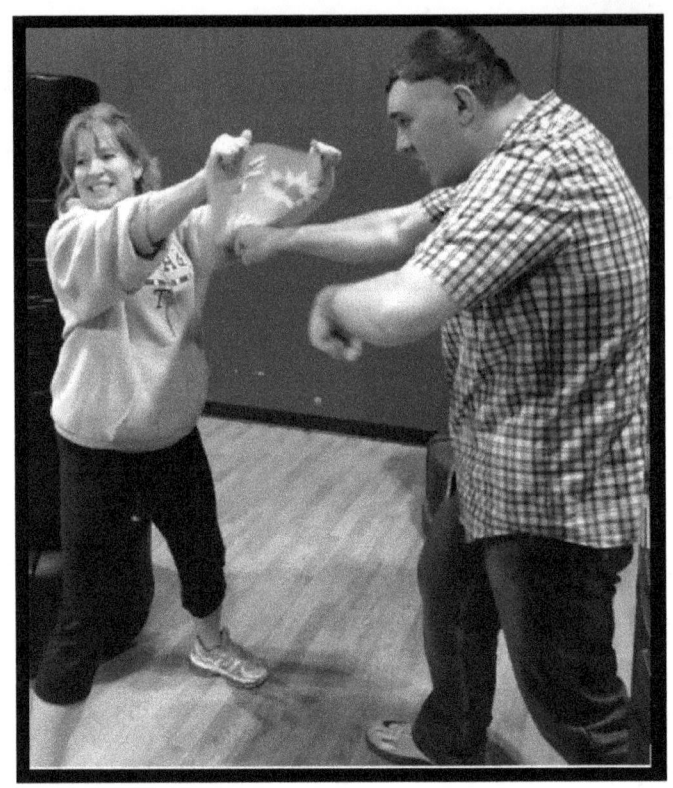

PAS FITNESS
CIRCUIT TRAINING
PHASE I

In Pas Fitness training, we want to work balance, ability, stability, better movement, better posture and confidence! To do all these great things, it is always wise to keep your routine fun and challenging.

There are THREE workouts provided for you:

•Pas Fitness Target – Duration: 2-3 times per week

With the Pas Fitness Circuit Training program, we are complimenting those things you worked on with the target and will build better core strength, better balance and better agility! Here we go…

You will need hand weights (3 to 5 pounds), one 10-pound weight, a chair and water!

Warm-up (three to five minutes)

- Jabs
- Squats with jabs
- Invisible punching bag

> • Those squats with the jabs can be very small if needed. If you cannot squat well, just make small squat motions – always be comfortable. You can do this!
> • If you are seated, attempt to raise alternate legs (even just a half inch if that is what you can do) with each punch.

Chair Squats – don't panic! You can do this. Re-read how to squat in the chapter on how to move. If you need an assisted squat, this is what you do:
= 3 sets/12 reps

Standing Kicks and Balance Holds

Stand behind your chair!

Lateral Leg Raise

Keep your back straight and chin up. Do not fold over the chair. With your foot parallel to the floor (sideways), slowly raise your leg up and down again but do not allow your leg to rest – do not set your foot on the floor.

Advanced: Take your hands off the back of your chair if you think you can test your balance. Only do this if you feel confident in your abilities.

- Lateral Leg Raise (left side)
- Lateral Leg Raise (right side)
- Lateral Leg Raise (left side)
- Lateral Leg Raise (right side)
- Lateral Leg Raise (left side)
- Lateral Leg Raise (right side)

=16 reps

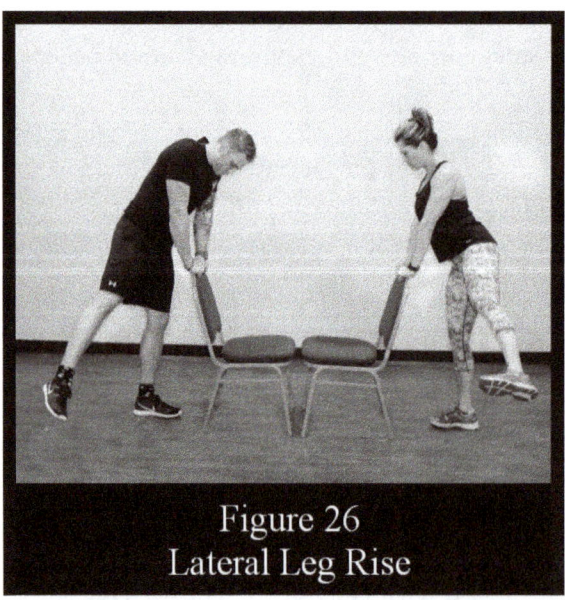

Figure 26
Lateral Leg Rise

In Figure 26, both Micah and Dionne are using the chair for the lateral leg raise but note how Dionne is using the chair for minimal balance only. Her back is straight and her raised leg is controlled and strong. Then, note how Micah is leaning heavily on the chair. In doing so, he's lost his posture and control of the raised leg – he is slumped forward (gorilla back!) and his leg is slightly behind him, foot relaxed.

In comparison, Dionne's leg is out to the side and her foot is flexed.

Calf Raises

Standing behind the chair, raise up as high as you can on your toes. As you come down, do NOT allow your heels to touch the floor. Just as your heels are about to touch the floor, raise back up again. You will feel a burn in the calf muscles and that sensation may travel up your legs. Wow! That is a wonderful way to wake up all those muscles and build strong ankles.

= 20 reps for 3 sets

Donkey Kick

Keep your back straight and stand tall. Feet centered behind the chair, slowly lift one leg behind you. Do not bend that leg! Slowly lift it, hold, then set it down but do not rest the foot on the floor. Repeat.

- Donkey Kick (left leg)
- Donkey Kick (right leg)
- Donkey Kick (left leg)
- Donkey Kick (right leg)
- Donkey Kick (left leg)
- Donkey Kick (right leg)

= 16 reps

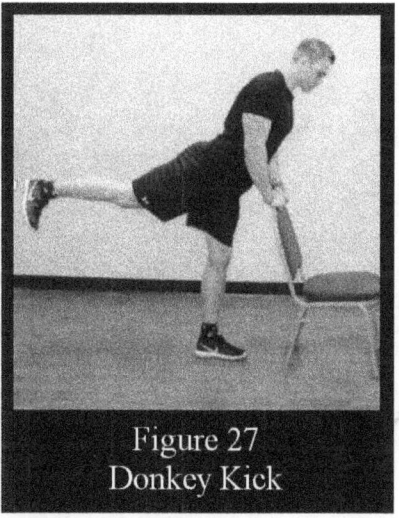

Figure 27
Donkey Kick

Goblet Squat

Get your weight.

Form is very important here. Holding the weight (Beginners: use the light weights. For stronger athletes, you may pick up the 10-pound weight) between both hands, just under your chin so that your head is up (good position for your back) and you squat down as low as you can, come back up until your legs are almost straight…then back down again. Because you have an added weight, be sure you are not tipping forward and you are back on your heels, weight over heels and hips.
= 12 reps

Superman – On the Floor or Standing with a Chair

You choose! You know what is best for you.

On the Floor

This is a great lower back exercise.

Full Superman

Lying on your stomach, raise up both legs and arms off the floor. Try to get the tops of your thighs off the floor for full extension. Chin is up. Hold. Then relax after a 10, 15, 20, or 30 second hold. Start again.

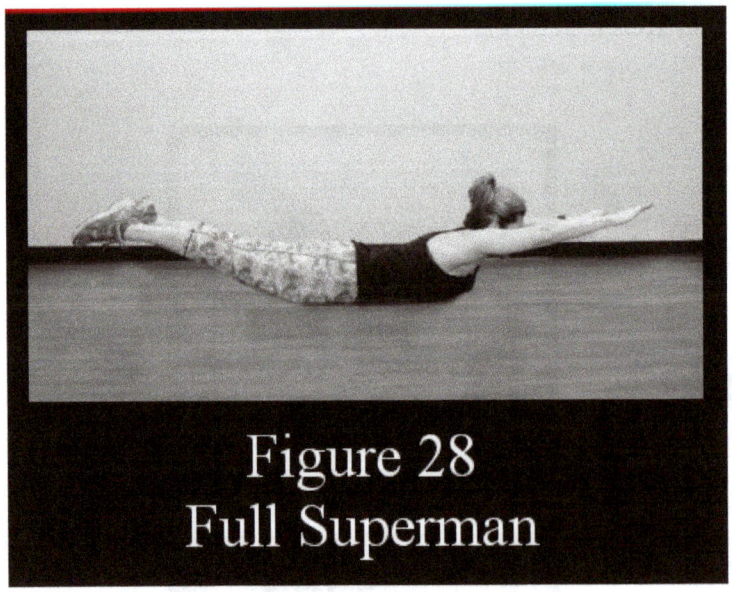

Figure 28
Full Superman

Half-Superman

On the Half-Superman, you are still on your stomach. Raise your left arm and right leg at the same time. Do NOT bend either leg or arm. Raise up. Chin up. Try to get the top of your thigh off of the floor and hold. Relax. Switch sides.

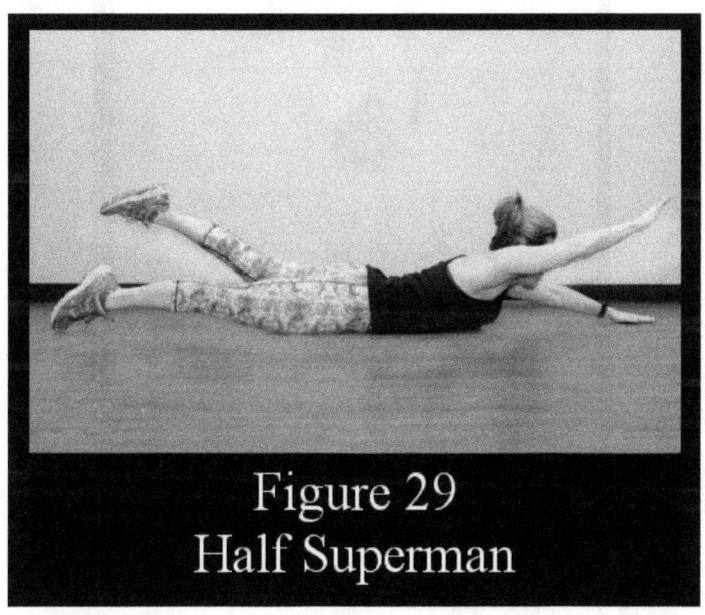

Figure 29
Half Superman

Other side – Raise your right arm and left leg and hold.

On a Chair

Half-Superman

Standing behind the chair, you are going to extend out and fly just like Superman. Let's start with the left side. Raise and extend your left hand forward. Next, extend out your right leg (do not bend it!) and hold.
Other side – Raise your right arm and extend that left leg. Chin is up. Back is straight and strong. Hold.

= 15 second hold each side for 3 sets

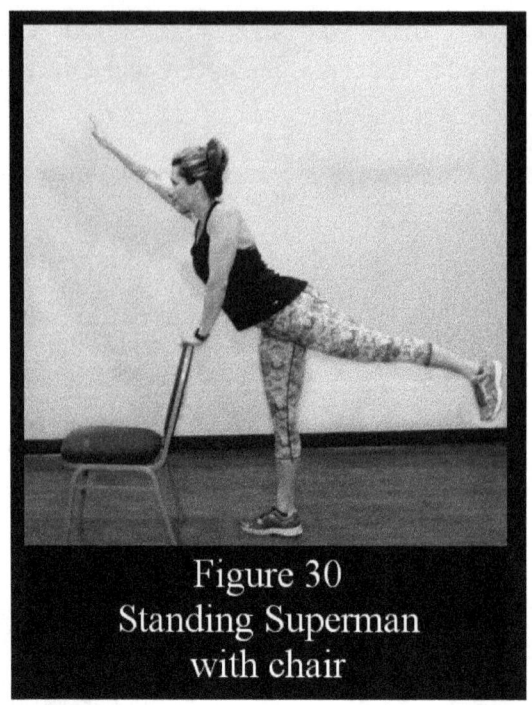

Figure 30
Standing Superman
with chair

Lower Abdominals/Feet on the Floor (Bridge)

If you are able to be on the floor – stay right there!

On the Floor – Bridge

Lying prone on the floor, pull your knees up and then place your feet flat on the floor about hip width apart, and your arms to your sides. Exhale as you push up and lift your hips all the way up toward the ceiling and hold for a second, then slowly lower to the ground. This is NOT a fast exercise. Take your time. The higher you raise your hips, the more you will feel the work in your lower abdominals, hips and legs.

= 15 second hold each side for 3 sets

On the Chair – Lower Abs

On the chair, it is not quite the same exercise but you will work those lower abs, hips and legs. Your focus is to keep your feet flat on the ground at all times. Do not let the feet come up. Sitting sideways in your chair, hold the side of the chair if you need support. Remember – safety first.

Slowly extend out, doing a reverse sit up. Slowly come up. You will feel your abdominal wall (muscles) shaking and you will want to raise those feet up but fight the urge and make your lower abdominal muscles work!

= 16 nice slow reps

Knee-to-Chest Kickout – On the Floor or Standing with a Chair

On the Floor

On your hands and knees on a padded mat on the floor, make sure your knees are just below your hips and your hands are directly under your shoulders. This is a very good position and not too much pressure on your hips, shoulder or elbow joints.

Draw your left knee up toward your chest and then gently push it back (like a donkey kick) straight out behind you. Your goal is to have your ankle/foot as high as your hip/bottom. Pull it back in. This is one repetition.

Be careful not to start swinging the leg and allowing your back to sway and roll out. Keep your back still and strong.

Other side – Right knee draws up toward your chest, then push it back, nice and high. Keep your back still and strong.

= 16 reps

On a Chair

Knee-to-Chest

Standing behind the chair, extend your arms out while holding on to the chair and raise up a knee (between your arms) toward your chest and kick it back. Again, be sure to keep your back still. Do not swing the leg so much that your back is sway and/or folding over the chair. Stand tall!

= 16 reps

Hip Circles – On the Floor or Standing with a Chair

On the Floor

On your hands and knees, raise your left leg and keep it bent. Imagine what a dog looks like when he urinates on a fire hydrant. Sorry! It is the best visual I can offer. After 20 years of teaching this, each time a new person does this exercise they always say, "We should call this the fire hydrant!"

Raise up that left leg and pulling the knee toward your chest, lift it and make a big circle motion (counter clockwise) until you complete one large circle. The larger you make the circle, the more of the hip and glutes you are working so go big! One circle is one repetition.

= 16 reps

Raise the right leg and make the same big circles

= 16 reps

Standing with Chair

Standing tall behind the chair, the idea is the same only you will work more to raise the knee up toward your shoulder and make your big circle motion that way. The bigger the circle, the more you are working the hip and glutes but because you are standing, you are also working the opposite leg and lower back as well. Stand tall and strong and do not sway as you make the circular movements.

Repeat on other side
= 16 reps

Cross-Abs and Balance – Standing or on the Chair

You have two choices here. Because many have bad knees or poor balance, you may have to work up to this and may want to stand. Let's start with the standing position:

Standing Cross-Abs and Balance

Standing behind your chair, raise your left knee upward and inward at the same time you bring down your right elbow until left knee and right elbow meet. When elbow and knee touch (or come close), extend both leg and arm outward – left foot out sideways to the floor and out to the side and right hand upward and out toward the ceiling. Think about making a star pattern.

It is very important to hold a good, strong back position here. Do not fold over the chair or drop your head. Stand tall. Be strong.
= 16 reps

Switch sides. Remember you may get tired and begin to roll out your back and fold inward. Stay strong. Bring the right knee upward and up to the chest to meet your left elbow. Stretch out.
= 16 reps.

Cross-Abs and Balance on the Chair

On your hands and knees ON THE CHAIR, you are going to really challenge your core strength and balance. Be sure that you are able to do this movement without falling. You know what you can do.

At the same time, extend your left leg and right arm straight out, then draw them in and touch your right elbow to left knee, hold, and stretch back out again. Got it? Repeat. You will feel your entire body shake as you struggle to work the entire core of your being.
= 16 reps

Switch sides. Raise right leg and left arm. Touch knee to elbow and stretch out again.
= 16 reps

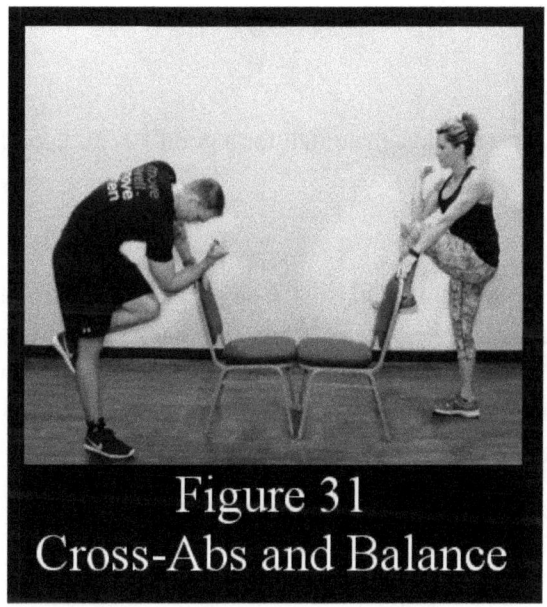

Figure 31
Cross-Abs and Balance

Note how Micah has collapsed forward. His head is dropped and his form is not controlled. Dionne, however, is standing tall and strong.

    Good job!!
    Let's cool down.

Shoulder Shrugs

    Pinch up the shoulders and hold for five seconds. Release and exhale. Ahhh! Repeat.
                  = 5 times

Shoulder Shrugs – rolling forward

    Roll your shoulders forward with big circles but keep your back straight, head held high.
                  = 5 times

Shoulder Shrugs – rolling backwards

    Roll your shoulders backwards, also in big circles. Chin up, back straight.
    = 5 times

Straight Arm Stretch

    Extend your right arm out in front of you. Place your left hand behind your right elbow and gently pull the arm in toward you. This should feel good. Do not continue to pull inward if this does not feel good.

    Release.

    Stretch the other side.

                    = Hold each stretch for a good 10-20 seconds

Leg Stretch

    On this stretch, posture is everything! Do NOT be a gorilla! No rolled backs.

    So…whether you are standing or seated, pull your toes back toward your knee. Straighten your back. Do NOT reach for your toes. Everyone always reaches for the toes. It is unnecessary and also causes you to roll the back! Lift your chin and imagine you are directing everything toward the knees. Toes and chin are pulled to the knee. Feel that? Oh, yes! That is an excellent stretch that you will feel from your mid-calf all the way up the leg.

    Again – this is supposed to feel good.

Be A Chicken

    Oh, the glorious chicken!

    It is time to be nice to your back, to your knees, to your hips, and to your shoulders so let's be a chicken.

    Head up, chin up.

    Pull your shoulders back. Chest up. Create a nice straight (and strong) line for your back.

    Now bend your knees very slightly and poke your bottom out just a little.

    Can you imagine how a chicken walks?

    Stand up and try that again!

    And again!

Let's Go Bowling

    Let's start with the right side.

    Imagine you have a bowling ball in your hand. Bring it up toward you chin, then pull the imaginary ball back as your opposite leg (left) steps forward. Gently swing your bowling ball arm forward while performing a slight forward lunge. Nice job.

    Are you watching your back?

    Just as if you were really bowling, make sure your back is strong, abdominal muscles are tightened, chin is up, shoulders and back are NOT rounded.

                    = Bowl 3 strikes!

    Let's move to the left side.

    The ball is in your left hand so as you draw the imaginary ball back, step forward with your right leg. Slight lunge. Chin up, back straight and abs strong.

                    = Bowl 3 strikes!

Let's Play Some Ball

You did a lot of punching and hooks so let's make sure your back and shoulders are nice and loose. Imagine you are playing basketball. Dribble your imaginary ball three times then take a shot. Let your hand stay up in the air for a moment (just like the pro NBA stars!) and repeat.

= Take 3 shots!

Repeat on other side = Take 3 shots!

Most people quit before they get the full benefit of a great workout.
Don't cheat yourself! Pas Fitness

The Pas Fitness Circuit Workout:

Chair Squats				
Lateral Leg Raise-left side				
Lateral Leg Raise-rightt side				
Calf Raises				
Donkey Kick- left side				
Donkey Kick-right side				
Front Knee-Up-left side				
Front Knee-Up-right side				

Goblet Squat				
Superman-left side				
Superman-right side				
Lower Abs/Feet on Floor Bridge				

Knee-to-Chest Kickout-left				
Knee-to-Chest Kickout-right				
Hip Circle-left				
Hip Circle-right				
Cross-Abs & Balance-left				
Cross-Abs & Balance-right				
Cool Down/Stretch				

PAS FITNESS
STABILITY TRAINING
PHASE I

In Pas Fitness training, we want to work balance, ability, stability, better movement, better posture and confidence! To do all these great things, it is always wise to keep your routine fun and challenging. There are THREE workouts provided for you:

- Pas Fitness Target – Duration: 2-3 times per week
- Pas Fitness Circuit – Duration: 1 time per week
- Pas Fitness Stability – Duration: 1-2 times per week

With the Pas Fitness Stability Training program, it is important to gain strength but also to work on functional movement. As we develop muscle memory and repeat specific movement patterns, we can develop better and safer movements that will help decrease risks of falling or hurting ourselves while becoming stronger and more independent!

Let's do HALF WORK and HALF FUN!

For the Stability Training session, you will need a set of hand weights of 3 to 5 pounds (but you can always increase the weight), a chair, and the Pas Fitnessmat. Don't forget your water.

Let's do the work first!

One Armed Row

Placing same side hand and knee on the chair, make sure your back position is strong. Engage the abdominal muscles, chin is up, and make sure your back and shoulders are flat. This is important as you do not want to roll out the back.

With your right knee and right hand on the chair, allow the weight in your left hand to pull toward the floor. Now, row upward so that your elbow steers toward the ceiling. Chin is up, back is flat and strong. Slowly release and repeat.

= 16 reps

Placing the left knee and left hand on the chair, now raise your right arm, guiding the right elbow upward toward the ceiling. Your back is long and strong, abs engaged, chin is up.

= 16 reps

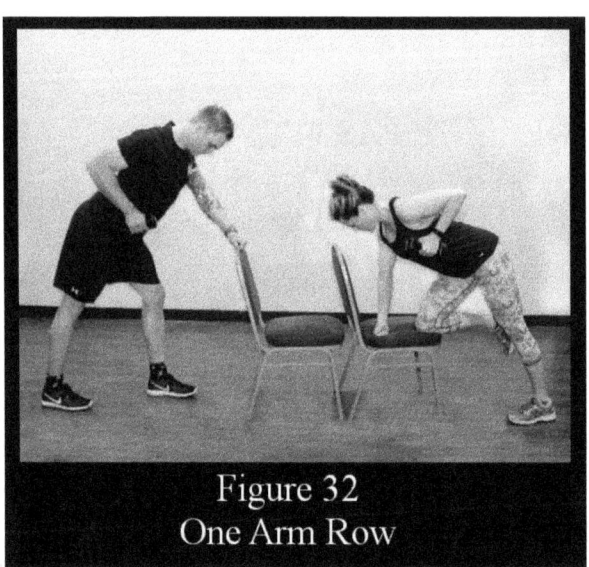

Figure 32
One Arm Row

Tricep Overhead

With a weight in your hand, raise your elbow toward the ceiling with the hand weight hanging behind your head, between your shoulder blades. Keep the raised elbow very, very still. The idea is to only work the muscle between your shoulder and elbow – the tricep. Slowly, raise the weight all the way up toward the ceiling – extending that arm, then lower it again, down between your shoulder blades. Do not rush this movement. It isolates that muscle behind your arm, near your armpit.

= 16 reps

Bicep Curls

Standing (or sitting) tall, hold both weights in your hands and keep your chin up. With this strong posture, alternate hands and slowly curl the weight up toward our body, keeping the palm of your hand turned inward to your body as you do.

Be sure not to allow your body to swing as you perform these bicep curls. Stand perfectly still. Be strong.

= 16 reps

Front Lateral Raises

Palm down, holding the weight, slowly raise your arms in front of you to be level with your shoulder. Pause, bring the weight back down. Again, this is not a fast motion but nice and slow to isolate the muscles. You should feel a burning sensation in your shoulders as you do this but you are also working your back, arms and abs!

= 16 reps

Overhead Press

Holding the weight with your palm facing outward, raise the weights to your shoulders. Standing tall, keep your head up and abdominal muscles engaged. Press the weights up to the ceiling and back down to your shoulder. Control each movement and make sure not to sway or bend forward.

= 16 reps

Push-Ups – On the Floor or Standing Against the Wall

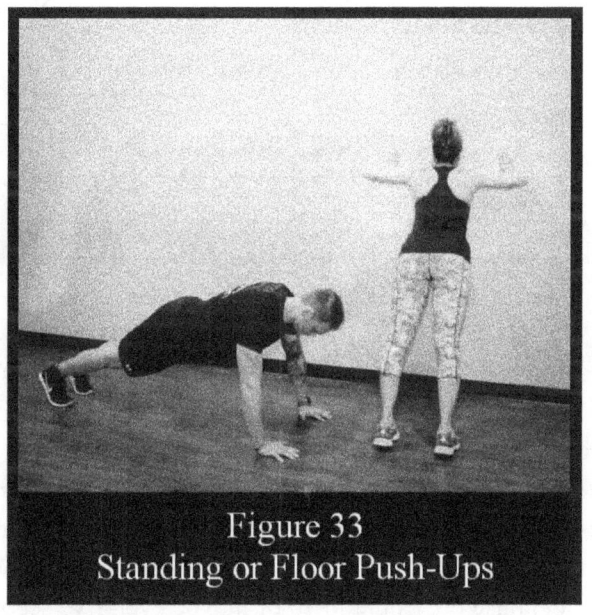

Figure 33
Standing or Floor Push-Ups

On the Floor

Begin lying face down on the floor. Place your feet shoulder width apart and hands measured on the side of your face so that your thumbs are almost even with your chin. This is very important: Imagine that your back and hips cannot bend but are straight as a board. Make sure that when you "push up" you rise in one straight unit.

Modified: You may perform these push-ups on your knees.
Advanced: Close the width of your feet. The narrower the stance, the more you challenge your core.

= 30 seconds

Your goal is to continue the push-up activity for 30 full seconds if you can and you will do three sets. If you cannot do 30 seconds, however, do not worry! You will get stronger over time. Write down how many seconds you were able to do continued push-ups.

Standing Pushups

The principle is the same. Standing with your feet shoulder width apart, stand approximately one foot from the wall. Remember that all people are different so you can adjust to the length of your arms. The further you are from the wall, the more challenging it will be. The closer you are to the wall, the easier it is.

Place your hands on the wall, thumbs level to where your chin will be as you do the push-up against the wall, shoulder width apart. Keep your feet flat on the floor as you dip in and move with control. Your back is straight. Do not bend forward and cheat that push-up.

Planks – Standing Planks or on the Floor

On the Floor

Your traditional plank is on the floor and is one of the best ways to build great abdominal and back muscles. Here's how:

Lying on the floor, place your feet about hip to shoulder width apart (like the push-up, the closer your feet are together, the more challenging this exercise becomes), and put your elbows just below your shoulders.

Raise up so that your entire body is as stiff and strong as a board! Do NOT poke your bottom up into the air.

Can't do a plank? Here is how to learn:

The biggest mistake people make with planks is they bend and raise their bottom higher than the rest of the body. Sure – it is easier that way but your abs never really get stronger. As you poke your bottom into the air, you are putting more weight on your feet and shoulders. You WANT to work the abs so…stay straight as a board and raise up. Count to 10 or maybe even five seconds if that is all you can do, ease back down to the floor, take a deep breath and try again.My students who are learning to do a GOOD plank will sometimes go back down on the floor five, six, even seven times in a 20 second hold and that is okay! That is how you learn and how you grow stronger.

= 20 second hold

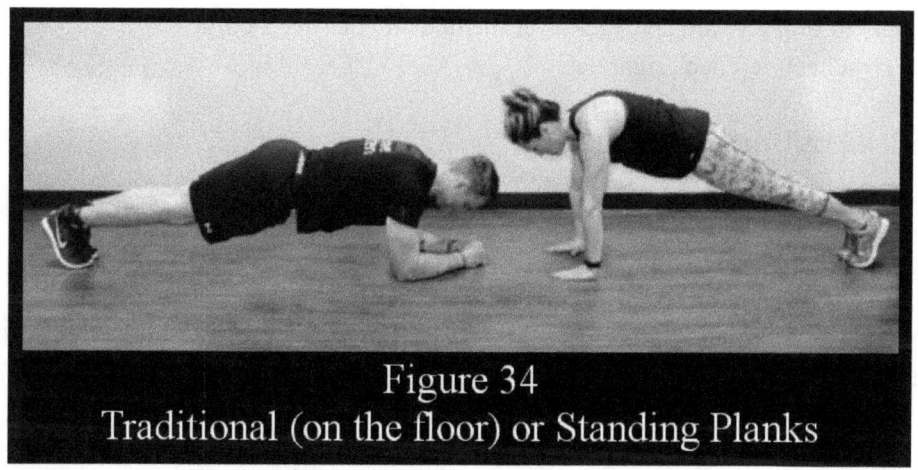
Figure 34
Traditional (on the floor) or Standing Planks

Standing Plank

Stand against the wall and place your forearms against the wall so that your elbows are almost as high as your shoulders. If you have bad shoulders, you can lower the arms to comfort.

Standing shoulder width apart, back your feet far enough away from the wall so that you are a perfect slant into the wall and hold. Practice controlled breathing and make sure your back is strong.

Pas Fitness Four Square

Using the Pas Fitness mat, it is time to work coordination, cognitive skills (thinking), agility and stability.

Step Over the Puddle – On Your Toes

Just as you would in real life, you are going to step over the line (pretend it is a puddle) and land gently on the ball of your foot.

Stand in one of the squares and starting with your right foot, step over first with your right foot, then your left, then step back again – first with the right foot and then the left. Stay on the ball of your feet. Do not set the heel down.

= 20 seconds

Repeat the movement pattern but this time, start with your left foot. Do not be surprised if you are more coordinated on one side than the other.

= 20 seconds

Heels Only

Just as you did with Over the Puddle, stand in a square and prepare to step over the line. Try not to step on the line itself. This time, however, you are rocked back on your heels. Pull your toes up toward the ceiling and try to step forward and back over the line on your heels only.

Left heel, right heel; left heel, right heel.
= 20 seconds
Right heel, left heel; right heel, left heel
= 20 seconds

Four Square – The Numbers Game

Okay – here we go. When you perform these steps, move quickly. The idea is to work your cardio but coordination as well. Ahhh, but you know what is the hardest? Just remembering the numbers.

1-2-4 Step

Starting with both feet in the #1 box, you will then either step or hop to box #2, then #4, and back to #1 again. Move as quickly as you can. Have someone count for you and see how many times you can complete a 1-2-4 circle patterns in 20 seconds!

3-4-2 Step

Starting with both feet in the #3 box, you are now going to move in the opposite direction. Either stepping or hopping, move quickly to box #4 and then to #2. Go around and around and try to count how many times you can complete a circle in 20 seconds. Be sure not to step on the lines!

1-4 Step

Start in box #1. Either step or hop between boxes #1 and #4. On this one, be sure to keep your hips forward so that you are moving laterally (side to side). It is very common to move your body sideways as you go faster and faster. Keep your body facing forward as you move between the two boxes. See how many times you can complete with in 20 seconds.

3-2 Step

Start in box #3. Either step or hop between boxes #3 and #2. On this one, be sure to keep your hips forward so that you are moving laterally (side to side). It is very common to move your body sideways as you go faster and faster. Keep your body facing forward as you move between the two boxes. See how many times you can complete with in 20 seconds.

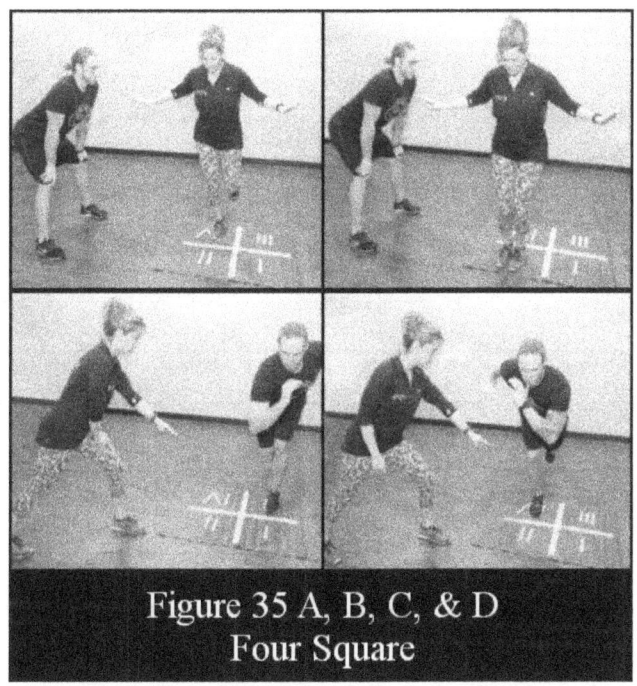

Figure 35 A, B, C, & D
Four Square

TRY THIS!

The Numbers Game!

Get a partner and challenge him or her to a real puzzler!
Have your buddy stand in the box. Time your buddy as you call out numbers in any random order. There are only four numbers so it can't be that hard, right?
Oh, it is hard!
Call out a series of numbers and you can speed up or slow down as you call the numbers. Your partner must try to land on those numbers as you call them out…but do not be too hard because you have to go next.

The PAS Fitness Stability Wokout

The Work				
One-Armed Rows-left side				
One-Armed Rows-right side				
Tricep Overhead-left side				
Tricep Overhead-right side				
Bicep Curls-left side				
Bicep Curls-right side				
Lateral Raise-together				
Overhead Press-left side				
Overhead Press-right side				
Push-ups-wall or floor				
Plank-wall of floor				

Now the Fun Begins...				
Step Over the Puddle-left side				
Step Over the Puddle-right side				
Heels Only-left side				
Heels Only-right side				
Four Square				
1-2-4 Repeat!				
3-4-2 Repeat!				
1-4 Repeat!				
2-3 Repeat!				

FINAL THOUGHTS

Pas Fitness is not just a whimsical workout that seemed fun because we can punch and kick, and be loud. Pas Fitness is a well-designed program that became part of a data-based research at the Occupational Therapy Department of Navarro College and within a Master's program at Tarleton State University's kinesiology department. The design was as following:

HYPOTHESIS

A fitness program designed for functional and developmental movement with cognitive tasks greatly improves the physical and behavioral skills of those living with disabilities. If implemented, the special needs community would benefit physically, socially, and medically.

OBJECTIVES OF THE STUDY
GENERAL OBJECTIVES
- To improve overall health for the special needs community and help them gain a sense of independence.
- Illustrate how the most basic functional movements can promote better physical and cognitive health.
- Outline a safe and effective fitness program to the special needs community.
- Offer Pas Fitness to the international fitness community for all trainers and facilities to adopt.
- Create an affordable, successful program to ensure confidence, promote better health.

SPECIFIC OBJECTIVES
- Assist student with cognitive skills, such as learning "left" from "right," and following basic directions or cues in a fitness class.
- Promoting individual health.
- Teaching students about their own bodies; create a program that encourages students to understand and appreciate their own bodies, such as naming major muscle groups.

-Teaching the value of self-worth and self-esteem.

After 12 weeks of working with students, the findings were undeniable.

SUMMARY FINDINGS

Following the 12-week study in which participants were assessed on physical abilities, as well as behavioral and social capabilities based on a regimented fitness course, the findings are:

1. How the study impacted the subjects, all of whom have a wide variety of disabilities, ranging from physical and/or mental and emotional:

>Every participant in the study improved in the areas of balance, agility, strength, independence, core, and stability. Forty-four percent (44%) of the physically disabled adults moved from scores of a 1 and/or 2 (meaning that the subjects were unwilling or unable to complete a physical task) to a score that reflected some level of independence and better strength and balance. All participants told their examiners they felt stronger; all participant asked to continue with the training program.
>
>The study finds a direct correlation between the improved scores of cross-pattern physical tasks and multi-directional cues to the significant improvement in the behavioral scores of the subjects, thus reinforcing the need to introduce multi-functional movements and cognitive skills in a physical program.

2. Environmental factors:

>The research shows that when the subjects continued with a structured program they were better able to take direction and discern between outside influences, such as noise or movement, and what was happening in their own classroom environment. As each subject excelled in the study, examiners noted that the subjects learned to stay on task or remain engaged with whomever they were working with rather than letting outside noise or activity distract them.

3. Confidence:

>The level of raised or secured confidence most surprised the examiners in this study. Subjects who previously would not allow themselves to be touched were offering high-fives; subjects who never spoke or would only look at that ground were engaging in conversation and held eye contact. All subjects reportedly were happier, more talkative, and willing to engage conversations with people not part of the study. All the subjects were willing to adapt and learn new exercises and material, including names of the human anatomy, distinguishing "left" from "right," and counting. There were some marked improvements with scores of 1 or 2 in week 1 that moved to a 4 or 5 in Week 12.

4. Behavior and social conditioning:

>As with the physical assessment results, all the subjects who scored a 1 or 2 (meaning the unwillingness or inability to respond appropriately to behavioral or social cues), moved

to a 3 or higher score. Subjects exhibited increased behaviors of responsibility and communication. The most unexpected but positive results noted by the examiners was the bond formed between the subjects. In no part of the study was there a section for monitoring teamwork or cheering for other participants in the study yet by mid-term, individuals were waiting for and/or cheering on others in the study to perform a task.

CONCLUSION

Based on the results of the study, the examiners and research team have determined that a regimented fitness program, specifically designed to improve functional movement and encourage problem-solving through directional patterns, core and stability tasks, greatly improves the overall health of those with special needs. Subjects who entered the study using assistive devices, such as walkers, canes, and leg braces, gained new independence. Those chair bound improved in range of motion in the upper body, and one subject excelled from limited mobility and a reliance on walkers to complete independence and the ability to get down on the ground and get up again without assistance. But the greatest improvements were made behaviorally and socially. Those who participated in the study became more socially aware, more confident, less fearful of new tasks or challenges, and displayed an eagerness to learn. For those young adults who could not count beyond "10" and were aware that others could, learning to count to "20" and/or discerning between their left and right hand created a notable change in their behavior among the examiners, researchers, peers, even fellow members of the gym and college facility.

For a full review of the study, please find it online: Better Function with Pas Fitness: A Study of Statistical Techniques Applied to Developmental and Physical Health in the Special Needs Community by Alexandra Allred.

The end result is just what we hoped for: Pas Fitness is for everyone!

KNOW THIS: These are big workouts and you used all your muscles. If you cannot complete the entire workout that is OKAY! I tell all my classes, from beginners to the very advanced, from college students to senior citizens, the goal to working out is to grow, get stronger, and feel good. Do what you can, mark down your successes. By marking down what you can do, you will also be able to see your own personal growth. Perhaps today you are only able to do half (or less) of the workout. That is okay! But write down what you did and stick with it. Soon enough, you will get stronger. You will punch and kick harder. You will punch and kick faster. You will have better balance.

Do you remember when you were asked, "Are you an athlete?" Remember this: When you work out and give it all that you have, when you think 'I can do no more,' when you are tired but also proud of what you did…you ARE an athlete. This is the experience that every Olympian, every professional athlete, every marathon runner, every CrossFit athlete, every martial artist, and every kickboxer has after a great session.

Be proud of yourself.
Be determined to get stronger.
Pas Fitness

ABOUT THE TEAM

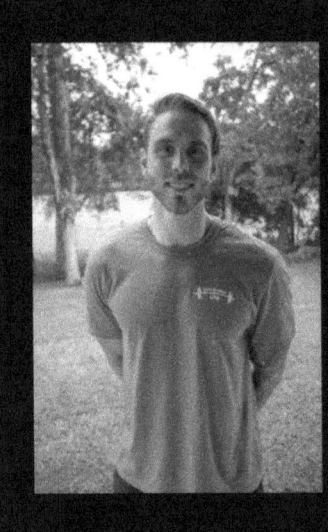

Micah Stewart

As the lead instructor at Main Street Gym, Micah has been more than a leader to members and staff. Micah is our resident expert on functional and corrective movement, holding an array of certifications, yet continues his education in kinesiology so he can continue to "drop knowledge" on those around him. Strong in faith, friends, and family, Micah also donates his time to working with those with disabilities.

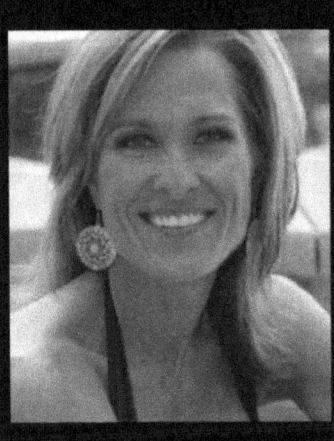

Dionne Zschiesche

The mother of three grown sons (and a grandmother!), Dionne is also a former fitness competitor, nationally ranked in the Masters Bikini Division.

Dionne Has gone on to train and help countless others in the fitness industry but may be best known for her huge heart.

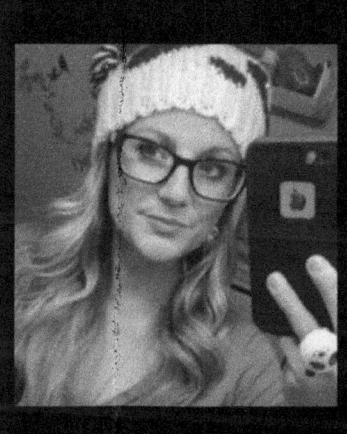

Amanda Sue
Our Photographer

Not only is she a talented photographer but Amanda Sue is an extremely popular yoga instructor, teaching all levels and always pushing people toward greatness. Amanda once battled depression and understands the importance of wellness, being active, and feeling strong and accomplished.

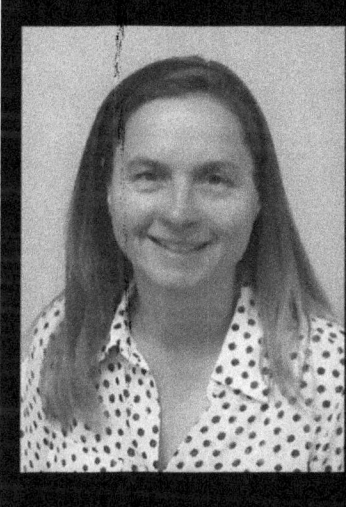

Melissa Boler
CEO, founder of Bridges Training Foundation

After 25 years in education, Melissa now counts herself lucky when she was assigned a special needs class. It changed her life and, in turn, she decided to change the world with the idea that everyone deserves the opprotunity for education, a job, and happiness. Melissa began a non-profit to help train young adults find a salaried job, purpouse in life, and a valued place in society. Without Melissa's passion, none of our work here would have been possible.

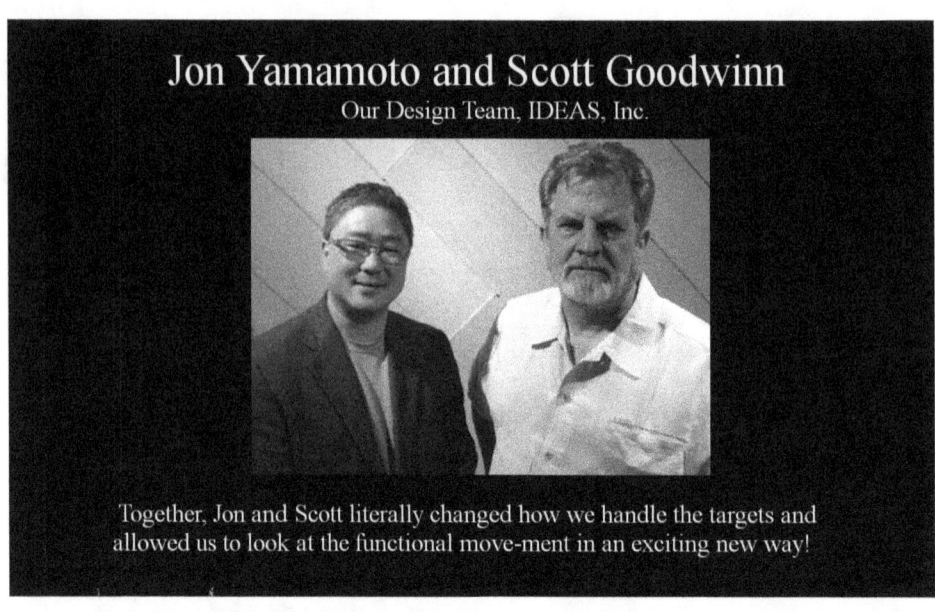

Jon Yamamoto and Scott Goodwinn
Our Design Team, IDEAS, Inc.

Together, Jon and Scott literally changed how we handle the targets and allowed us to look at the functional move-ment in an exciting new way!

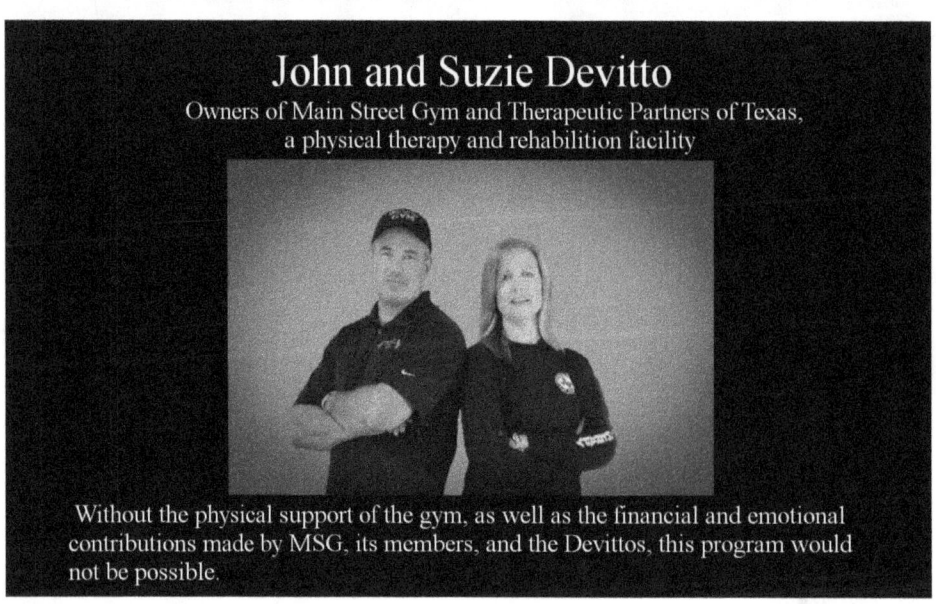

John and Suzie Devitto
Owners of Main Street Gym and Therapeutic Partners of Texas, a physical therapy and rehabilitation facility

Without the physical support of the gym, as well as the financial and emotional contributions made by MSG, its members, and the Devittos, this program would not be possible.

Our Team Motto:

We are all greater than that obstacle before us!

FIGURES

Figure 1 – Bicep curls (bad)
Figure 2 – Bicep curls (good)
Figure 3 – Lateral front raise (bad)
Figure 4 – Lateral front raise (good)
Figure 5 – Overhead press (bad)
Figure 6 – Overhead press (good)
Figure 7 – 1-2-1-2 Punches
Figure 8 – Front jab (good vs bad)
Figure 9A – Hook punch (good vs bad)
Figure 9B – Hook with the Target
Figure 10 – Upper cut (bad)
Figure 11 – Upper cut (good)
Figure 12A –Front kick, knee up
Figure 12B – Front kick, kicking
Figure 12C – Front kick with Micah, bad form
Figure 13A – Round kick, knee up
Figure 13B - Round kick, full extension
Figure 14A – Outside crescent kick (knee up)
Figure 14B - Outside crescent kick (the full kick)
Figure 15A – Hook kick (extension)
Figure 15B – Hook kick (the hook)
Figure 16 –   Chart on muscles and what they do:
        https://www.pinterest.com/source/endoszkop.com
Figure 17 –   Chart on skeletal and muscle development:
        https://www.pinterest.com/source/endoszkop.com
Figure 19A – the Gorilla, front
Figure 19B – the Gorilla, side view
Figure 20 –   the Chicken
Figure 21 – Chart of pounds per pressure on head and neck:
        http://www.theatlantic.com/health/archive/2014/11/what-texting-does-to-thespine/382890/
Figure 22 A and B – squats with a dowel and tape measurement
Figure 23A and B – squat (good vs bad)
Figure 24 A and B – squat (good vs bad)
Figure 25 A and B – chair squats (good vs bad)
Figure 26 – Lateral Leg Raise
Figure 27 – Donkey Kick
Figure 28 – Full Superman
Figure 29 – Half Superman
Figure 30 – Standing Superman (with chair)

Figure 31 – Cross-Abs and Balance
Figure 32 – One Arm Rows
Figure 33 – Standing or Floor Push-Ups
Figure 34 – Traditional (on the floor) or Standing Planks
Figure 35 a-d Four Square

RESOURCES

While there are hundreds and hundreds of wonderful organizations to help those with individual/special needs, Pas Fitness training recognizes 30 such organizations known for great community efforts, educational and training opportunities, resources for medical advice and/or rehabilitation, fitness and growth opportunities.

Bridges Training Foundation
www.bridgestf.org

What they offer: Bridges Training Foundation, LLC, is a nonprofit organization established with the primary goal of providing occupational and educational services to children and adults who have intellectual and developmental disabilities. Currently, Bridges is focused on working with adults ages 18+ to prepare and train them to enter the work force and become more independent through self-sustenance.
*This is a Texas non-profit only with long-term goals to offer national assistance.

Disabled American Veterans
www.DAV.org

What they offer: Dedicated to empowering veterans to lead high-quality lives with respect and dignity, DAV offers counseling, assistance in obtaining benefits, education the public about the needs of our veterans and how to transition back to civilian life.

Easter Seals
www.easterseals.com

What they offer: Resources for autism, seniors, children, adults, military and veterans, employment and training, medical rehabilitation, recreation, brain health.
Teams of therapists, teachers and other health professionals help each person overcome obstacles to independence and reach his or her personal goals. Easter Seals also includes families as active members of any therapy program, and offers the support families need.

Federation for Children with Special Needs
www.fcsn.org

What they offer: The Federation for Children with Special Needs (FCSN) provides information, support, and assistance to parents of children with disabilities, their professional partners, and their communities. They are committed to listening to and learning from families, and encouraging full participation in community life by all people, especially those with disabilities. FCSN believes that individual differences in people are a natural part of life, and that disabilities provide children and adults with unique perspectives, insights and abilities which contribute to the overall well-being of society.

Goodwill
www.goodwill.org

What they offer: Financial coaching, savings and loan support, tax preparation, education programs, community services, financial aid, transportation, after school programs, housing assistance, clothing assistance, medical rehabilitation.
Goodwill works to enhance the dignity and quality of life of individuals and families by strengthening communities, eliminating barriers to opportunity, and helping people in need reach their full potential through learning and the power of work.

Parents Helping Parents
www.php.com

What they offer: Support groups, family and community services, crisis support, early intervention, assistive technology services. Parents Helping Parents works with our community's most vulnerable populations – individuals with any special need and their families. This includes children of all ages and all backgrounds who have a need for special services due to any special need, including but not limited to illness, cancer, accidents, birth defects, neurological conditions, premature birth, learning or physical disabilities, mental health issues, and attention deficit (hyperactivity) disorder, to name a few.

Special Needs Alliance
www.specialneedsalliance.org

What they offer: Connection to attorneys in your area that practice disability and public benefits law, covering special needs trusts and wills, Medicare, SSI, estate and tax planning, personal injury, health care, financial planning, guardianships and conservatorships. The Special Needs Alliance (SNA) is a national, not for profit organization of attorneys dedicated to the practice of disability and public benefits law. Individuals with disabilities, their families and their advisors rely on the SNA to connect them with nearby attorneys who focus their practices in the disability law arena.

Special Olympics
www.specialolympics.org

What they offer: Real sports, building communities, youth activation, healthy lifestyle promotion, leadership, research. Our athletes find joy, confidence and fulfillment — on the playing field and in life. They also inspire people in their communities and elsewhere to open their hearts to a wider world of human talents and potential. Here's a slideshow showing the full spectrum of our activities.

The Arc
www.thearc.org

What they offer: Information and referral services, individual advocacy to address education, employment, health care and other concerns, self-advocacy initiatives, residential support, family support, employment programs, leisure and recreational programs. The Arc is the largest national community-based organization advocating for and serving people with intellectual and developmental disabilities and their families. We encompass all ages and more than 100 different diagnoses including autism, Down syndrome, Fragile X syndrome, and various other developmental disabilities.

Specialized Services

Autism
Autism Speaks
www.autismspeaks.org

Autism Society
www.Autism-society.org

National Autism Center
www.nationalautismcenter.org

Cerebral Palsy
Cerebral Palsy
www.cerebralpalsy.org

Cerebral Palsy Foundation
www.yourcpf.org

United Cerebral Palsy
www.ucp.org

Dementia and Alzheimer's Disease

Alzheimer's Association: Alzheimer's Disease and Dementia
www.alz.org

Alzheimer's Foundation of America
www.alzfdn.org

Dementia Society of America
www.dementiasoceity.org

Down Syndrome

Global Down Syndrome Foundation
www.globaldownsyndrome.org

National Down Syndrome Society
www.ndss.org

National Association for Down Syndrome
www.nads.org

Intellectual and Developmental Disabilities

American Association on Intellectual and Developmental Disabilities
www.aaidd.org

Association of Professional Developmental Disabilities Administrators
www.apdda.org

The Arc (for people with Intellectual and Developmental Disabilities)
www.thearc.org

Parkinson's Disease

American Parkinson Disease Association
www.apdaparkinson.org

National Parkinson Foundation
www.parkinson.org

Parkinson's Disease Foundation
www.pdf.org

Stroke

American Stroke Association
www.strokeassociation.org

National Stroke Association
www.stroke.org

World Stroke Organization

www.world-stroke.org

ABOUT THE AUTHOR

Alexandra Allred began her martial arts career in 1983, studying under Master Jhoon Rhee, Ernie Reyes, and some of the top martial artists in the nation, including Master Jim Choate, with whom Allred was honored with a 4th Degree Black Belt. Master Choate was one of the first martial artists responsible for demanding proper safety gear for fighters in the ring and helped change the course of history in tournament fighting.

But Allred had already carved her own history in the sports world, becoming the first champion named to the first ever U.S. women's bobsled team in 1994. Allred won U.S. Nationals, was named Athlete of the Year by the United States Olympic Committee for her sport, and was also pregnant. Following her work with renowned researcher of reproductive biology at Case Western Reserve University, Dr. James Clapp, III., Allred's data was used by the United States and International Olympic Committees in regards to athlete and safety performance for pregnant athletes. Allred later became a "pregnancy expert" with a number of national publications and websites.[17]

Allred is the author of dozens on books on wellness, fitness, sports as well as fiction. Allred continues to lecture on public health, environmental issues, and fitness on a national forum and is a new champion for special needs with Pas Fitness.

---

[17] www.pregnancy.org/questions/fitnessexpert

www.ingramcontent.com/pod-product-compliance
Lightning Source LLC
Chambersburg PA
CBHW080215040426
42333CB00044B/2700